"How To Survive After Open Heart Surgery For a Meat and Potatoes Guy."

"How To Survive After Open Heart Surgery For a Meat and Potatoes Guy."

Ralph G. Nigh

A SURVIVOR

AND OVER COMER

authorHOUSE®

AuthorHouse™
1663 Liberty Drive
Bloomington, IN 47403
www.authorhouse.com
Phone: 1-800-839-8640

First published by AuthorHouse   02/22/2012

ISBN: 978-1-4634-2790-0 (sc)
ISBN: 978-1-4634-2789-4 (ebk)

Library of Congress Control Number: 2011910758

Printed in the United States of America

Dedicated to my Grandchildren

Trevor Dunn

Courtney Routhe

Alvin (James) James Goehring IV

Taylor Rene Nigh

Julieanne Nora Marie Goehring

Caden Nicholas Nigh

Delaney Marie Nigh

Cody Michael Nigh

Brandon Lane Lathum

Braden Krull

Sienna Krull

Sophie Krull

Saylor Nigh

Without them this book would not be possible, because they are my inspiration to live, and my best friends. I want to see them grow-up.

Prologue

My name is Ralph G. Nigh. I was born in St. Joseph, Missouri on a snowy January 20th in 1949. I got hit in the temple with a rock at age two, shot by a friend at age 14. I was in my best friends care when he wrapped it around a telephone pole when I was 15 and I sawed my finger in half at age 16. I fell from my horse at age 58 and received a Subdural

Hematoma and I have had 3 open heart surgeries. I have also had 5 stints and 4 bypasses. I survived all that.

I graduated Lafayette High School in June 1967. I then enlisted in The United States Marine Corps, and soon found myself I Vietnam. I survived 4 different offensives including the 1968 Tet Offensive, where I was blown up and set on fire. I volunteered for Operation Desert Storm, JTF GTMO, where I almost drown and Operation Joint Endeavor.

I have 4 sons and a daughter and in the late 80's and early 90's I played full contact football with high school seniors without pads or helmets in all kinds of weather including rain, snow, sleet and ice. We survived.

I served as a Correction Officer at Western Missouri Correction Center in Cameron, MO. I also served as a Transportation Officer at the Maryville, MO and later as a SGT and Cert Team Officer with the Maryville Treatment Center MO. Dept Of Corrections.

In March of 2000, I went on Active Duty with the United States Army Chaplains Corps at Fort Hunter Liggett, California. In April of 2001 I took leave and worked as a Platoon Sergeant in the movie "WE WERE SOLDIERS", Mel Gibson and Sam Elliot, where I jumped out of helicopters, ran up and down mountains and crawled up and down checking lines all night for a week. I have been very active in all my life, and never backed away from a challenge.

I survived all that to learn on May 30th 2002 that I had 4 blocked arteries. On June 1st I had by-pass surgery. I survived the most difficult ordeal of my life, until August 29th of 2002 when I learned that I also had to have a bi-cusped aortic valve replaced. I had already missed 3 months of work and was that far behind. I asked the Dr. if he could wait until after the 1st of October so that I would have time to catch up and wouldn't be 6 months behind. I also need to close out the financial books, set up the new fund management system, and start the new physical year. He agreed. On the 7th day of October 2002 I went in for an aortic valve replacement.

In this book I will tell you how I survived the pain and cardiac diet. This will hopefully help some of you who are at risk of heart attack and have been told that you need to go on a reduced fat and low sodium diet. I will tell you meat and potatoes guys and gals how you can eat the 30 grams of fat diet without giving up all the foods you love like Pizza and burritos, chilly and many other dishes you love.

I have 12 grand children, who I plan to spend most of my time with after retirement. We are going to raise horses and be best friends. If not for the Drs., Nurses, Hospitals and the surgeries and the cardiac diet, I wouldn't be around to enjoy them.

CHAPTER I

THE DIAGNOSIS

THE DATE WAS DECEMBER 5th 1996 and I was working the night shift on a war fighter exercise at Fort Hood, Texas, it was about midnight and I felt these really strong chest pains. The First Sergeant saw me rubbing my chest, he asked, "What's wrong?" I answered, "I am having chest pains and I don't know why, but probably just heartburn." The Top said to SSG Alonzo "Take SSG Nigh to the Hospital."

SSG Alonzo rushed me to the Hospital that was only a few blocks away. When we walked in and told why we were there, they sprang into action. First they put me on an emergency room bed (if you can call that a bed, more like a table with sheets on it and wheels under it) and stuck Nitro Glycerin under my tongue (sub-lingual). The next step was to stick connectors to me with little snaps on them so they can hook up an EKG Machine (Electro Cardio Gram) to them. The Nitro did no good and the EKG showed nothing, so they admitted me to the Hospital for more tests.

Those of you who have been in the hospital on a cardiac diet know how tasteless the diets are, so here is your 1st tip. If you know that you are going into the hospital for cardiac testing take with you a blue 3 & 1/8th oz shaker of Morton Salt Substitute for salt free diets. It has an aftertaste if you put it in you hand and taste it that way. You can taste the salty taste, and when you put it on food the aftertaste goes away. You get a good salty taste that will make the cardiac diet a little more tolerable.

Next they did a stress test to see how my EKG reacted to stress. It took me over 30 minutes to get to the target heart rate they wanted and it showed nothing. Then, I was sent for CT (Computerized Tomography), which also showed nothing unusual.

After 3 days in the hospital at Fort Hood Texas I returned to my duty on the night shift in the War Fighter scenario with a bottle of Prilosec and was told that my chest pain was gastric. Since then I never had a problem physically doing anything that I wanted to do including running fast enough to beat many of the young people in my unit. On our semiannual Army Physical Fitness Test (APFT) and in January 1996 I turned 47 years old.

The Drs. have always asked has your Father, Mother, Sisters, Brothers, Aunts or Uncles ever had heart related problems. My answer always was (and had to be) no. It wasn't until I was in the Hospital after being cut open to have the triple bypass on June 1st 2002, that I realized that many things had different names medically in the 1920s and 1950s than they do today. I remembered that my Grandfather Nigh died of hardening of the arteries at the age of 70 and that my Grandfather Tritten had hardening of the arteries and died of a stroke at age 53, which is how old I was at the time of the surgery. Remember to think about your grand parents and the changes in terminology.

After completing my reserve training at FT. Hood I returned home to my house in Savannah, MO, and returned to work at the Maryville Treatment Center, MO Department of Corrections and on 15 February 1997 I had chest pains at work, while in the patrol car on perimeter patrol. I felt like I could drive to the hospital and notified the shift commander. The shift commander called the hospital and asked them to send out an ambulance. The ambulance came and when they decided to transport me to the hospital I said I couldn't pay for an ambulance. The shift commander LT. Burton said, "Don't worry about anything, the Department of Corrections will pay for it because you are at work and you don't have a choice in the matter." When the Superintendent (Prison Warden) received the bill he said they aren't paying for an ambulance ride for a personal illness. I then explained what had transpired and what LT Burton said. The Superintendent then said that if LT Burton would confirm that he said that, the Department would pay the bill. To date the bill still isn't paid, almost 7 years later. My point in bringing this up is don't trust anybody with you health or payment of your medical bills, cause when push comes to shove most people only wanted to give lip service and aren't going to get involved.

The Cardiologist at the hospital checked me out in the emergency room and after about 3 hours sent me back to work with an appointment with a Dr. at Northwest Missouri Cardiology for more extensive testing. When I arrived at his office he said that he was going to send me to the hospital for a cardiac stress test and an echo cardio gram. I went to the hospital and had the tests and was later told that they couldn't find anything wrong.

Soon my Dr. then said he was going to send me to a cardiologist in St. Joseph, Missouri to look a little deeper into the chest pains. The Cardiologist he sent me to was a young Cuban Dr. who seemed to have a lot on the ball he looked at the information from the test the other Drs. had done and said that he was going to order a stress echo. The other tests didn't show anything wrong and the gastric tests that I had taken didn't show that my stomach was that bad either. The Dr.

3

kept canceling the test because he had to go home to Cuba and to Florida a lot to visit relatives. After about 4 months of cancellations I received military orders to go to Ft. Dix, New Jersey for the summer for Active Duty Special Work. When I came back I got very busy and my chest pains didn't seem so bad, maybe I just learned to live with them and kept taking my Prilosec.

After returning from Fort Dix in September of 1997 I changed duties with the Missouri Department of Corrections and became transportation Officer, which was quite a change of pace from standing on the hard concrete all day watching the Inmates activities. Now transporting them to and from Dr. appointments and doing prisoner exchanges with other institutions and transporting them to and from funerals, county jails and court appearances. In April 1998 I was promoted to SGT and applied for the E-Squad, this was the department's version of the SWAT team or as some states call them the CERT team. I made it after taking a Physical fitness test and scoring the second highest score of anyone in this testing group.

In the ensuing months we had some very vigorous training, and as a SGT it was up to me to set the example for the junior officers, so I worked physical harder than many of the others. When fall came I was sent to Instructor training for Chemical Agents for the Department of Corrections. The third night after training my pager went off just after I got to bed. I got up and called in, we have an emergency situation at the Institution the control room SGT said you are to report to the E-Squad building as quickly as possible in camouflaged utilities. On the way in I listened to my scanner and had my flashers on moving as fast as legally possible. On the scanner I heard that there were hostages being held in medical.

Upon arrival at the Institution I grabbed my bulletproof vest and all of my equipment and we marched to the gate some officers drew weapons and surround the perimeter while my CERT team entered the institution and smartly moved in formation to the medical area. On arrival at the medical area we poised in the stairwell waiting for Intel reports. Finally we moved in and took down the hostage taker.

We then proceeded to the control center and drew weapons and took up positions with the rest of the E-Squad to search for the other two escapees. On the way to join the others there was a call over the radio to move to the west center of the perimeter, Man down. When we arrived at that location two officers had an inmate on the ground. The inmate was bleeding from wounds received from the razor ribbon wire when he climbed the fence. We quickly learned that only one more inmate was on the loose and outside. The wounded inmate was immediately taken to the hospital along with the two officers who found him and rendered first aide. The inmate was treated for his injuries and the officers where treated for blood exposure.

We set up a perimeter around the institution and began searching in a systematic manner. Daylight was beginning to pop up its head when we located the inmate in a brush pile, hidden under some boards in a hand-dug hole. All secure and all is well. We spent a couple of hours doing reports and listen to after action reviews this exercise was over.

I then proceeded to the university to attend the remainder of the chemical agents class. In all this I had no physical problems and kept up with kids half my age, something I have been doing with the U.S. Army since 1989.

My regular duties with the department of corrections had me serving as a housing unit SGT, Zone SGT and Visiting room SGT, jobs that would normally be held by 3 people. Even with all that additional stress I was being told that I was doing an outstanding job by all 3 of my supervisors. I was not feeling any adverse physical problems from the added stress.

In July 1999 my best friend, who was on active duty with the U.S. Army Reserve stationed at Ft. McCoy, Wisconsin, called me and said if I was still interested in active duty to get my packet in for it, now, as there were several positions coming open soon.

I followed Chucks instructions and sent my packet to the Full Time Support Management Team for consideration by the AGR (Active Guard Reserve) board for Active Duty. The AGR Board met in October and I was told in November that I had been accepted. In December SGM Burg called me from USARC to give me my options. He offered me several places I could go; the one that sounded the best was Ft. Hunter Liggett, CA, because it was warm year around. SGM Burg said you got it we will get your orders submitted quickly and we'll get you into the program as soon as possible. January rolled around and I was contacted by FTSMT and told the first class I could attend to get started would be 18 March 2000.

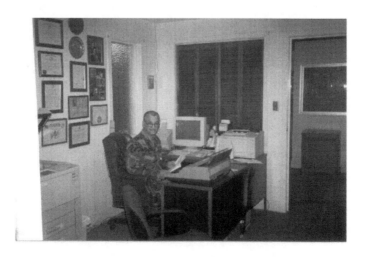

On 18 March 2000 I began my AGR career and soon arrived for duty at Ft. Liggett, CA. as the Installation Chapel NCOIC/Chaplain Assistant. My duties include physically maintaining the Chapel, Chapel administration, ministering to enlisted soldiers by listening to there problems and making referrals to the appropriate authority and make reports to the Chaplain including doing pre-counseling interviews for the Chaplain. My duties also included other duties as directed by the Chaplain.

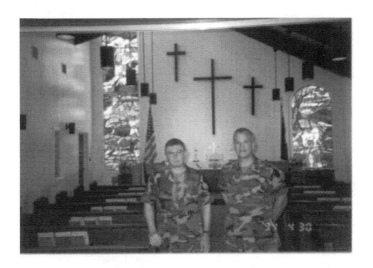

In June of 2000 I attended a school at Ft. Jackson, SC for Fund Clerk training. Upon returning I added Chapel Non-Appropriated fund clerk to my duties. I immediately was task with preparing the fund files from the past 1 ½ years for an audit at the end of August. By the time the auditor arrived, after only 2 weeks, the fund was in such good shape that we passed the audit/inspection with no discrepancies.

In January 2001 I attended a school at Fort Knox, KY to become an Equal Opportunity

Representative. This was another responsibility that was added to my duties when I became the Installation EOR. My duties were to hear complaints of sexual or racial harassment and take a report then make referral to the appropriate authority, such as the JAG, the Military Police, the Chaplain or the Equal Opportunity Advisor or other authorities as deemed appropriate.

In February 2001 I attended a special staff meeting to discuss plans for a movie that Mel Gibson's production company wanted to film at Ft. Hunter Liggett. Upon learning that I was a Vietnam veteran the production company became very interested in finding me a part in the movie. The filming started in late March. In April I took 2 weeks leave to play SFC Houston, one of the "Three War Men" who landed at Anzio with the 3rd Infantry Division and Jumped into Normandy on D-day with the 82nd Airborne, then

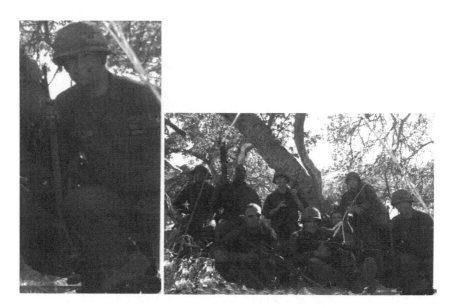

fought in Korea at Pork Chop Hill and is about to earn a second star for his Combat Infantry Badge. The Movie was a lot of work crawling up and down the lines in the dark, jumping out of helicopters and running up and down mountains. I learned that I could still keep up with the kids in combat and could still be a grunt. I was proud to have been in the only film made that got Vietnam Right.

The Morning of 11 September 2001 I woke up and turned to Good Day LA, as was part of my morning routine. Immediately I was shocked to see an airliner in one of the towers of the World Trade Center in New York City. My first thought was a tragic accident until I saw another plane coming around and crash into the other tower, I then new we were at war. I told my wife what was going on and took off for headquarters. When I arrived at headquarters the Installation Commander was the only one there and he said that he was calling a meeting at 0900 to set up emergency procedures. He said go home, have a good breakfast you may be vary busy by lunchtime.

We all converged on headquarters as 0900 rolled around and we met in the command conference room. I was assigned to help set up and work in the emergency operations center. I wound up working without any sleep for the next 48 hours. For the next 2 weeks I worked the 12 hour night shift in the emergency operations center from 2000 hundred hours (8 PM) to 0800 (8 AM) and attended the morning briefing at 0900 each day except Sunday when I worked all day at the chapel doing my regular duties. The stress levels got very high and after 2 weeks I started working back at my regular job except Thursday, Friday and Saturday when I worked with the Installation security with the Fort Hunter Liggett Police. Sundays were back at the chapel. Sometime in November we went back to regular duties when the California National Guard took over our Security functions.

In December 2001 I was having increased heartburn and went to the clinic on post and they told me that I should have my esophagus checked because GERDS can damage the esophagus enough to cause esophageal cancer. I went to the Navel hospital in Lemoore and had a camera put down my throat. The result was there was no cancer but I was put on Nexium to heal the Damage even though the Dr said it wasn't that bad.

In April 2002 I was coughing and having chest pains with a lot of head congestion. I went to the Clinic and talked to the medics they and the Physicians Assistant listened to my heart and lungs. They said they didn't hear anything wrong with my heart. My lungs were clear so they decided to do and EKG which they couldn't see anything wrong with my heart. Because my lungs were clear and I was having chest pains they decided to send me to Dr. Sinph at the Presidio of Monterey Military Health Clinic.

Dr. Sinph listened to my heart and ran an EKG, and couldn't hear or see anything wrong. Dr. Sinph decided that because of the chest pains that he would send me to a cardiologist. He then put me on a no Physical Training Profile from 30 April to 30 May, which is when my appointment was scheduled with Dr. Harlan Grogan at Central Coast Cardiology.

CHAPTER II

TRIPLE BYPASS

I DROVE TO SALINAS, ABOUT 80 miles away and walked into the Central Coast Cardiology office on 30 May 2002 for a Stress Test Cardiogram. When they took me into the EKG room I was told to sit on the table and the technician would hook me up to get a base line. He got me hooked up, ran a strip and said I don't like what I see lay down, I'm going to do and Echo.

Soon he said I don't like what I see I'll be right back. In a matter of seconds he returned with Dawn Tamagni Nurse Practitioner and he again moved the Eco stylist around on my chest. Nurse Tamagni then said I see what you mean. They sat me up and said "Mr. Nigh your heart isn't beating symmetrically" and she was going to talk to Dr. Grogan and would be right back. In a matter of moments she returned. Nurse Tamagni said she was going to get someone to take me in a wheel chair a block down and across the street to the emergency room.

Upon arrival at the emergency room of the Salinas Valley Memorial Hospital the nurses began hooking me up to cardiac monitors and putting in I.V.s. Soon the emergency room Dr came in an said asked if I was having any chest pain, to which I replied, "Just the pressure and heartburn that I have been feeling for the past 6 years. He then started and I.V. of saline and nitro glycerin.

After a half hour or so Dr. Grogan came in and said that he was going to send me up to the cardiac care center as soon as they had a room ready. Dr. Grogan then stated that in the morning at 7:30 they were going to take me into the cardiac catheter lab and do a heart catheter to get a good look at what the problem is. He said if they couldn't find any blockage they would pursue other avenues but if they found any blockage that they would try to do a balloon angioplasty to take care of the blockage. He also said that if they found blockage that was too bad that they would be able to do the balloon and would discuss my options as soon as I was coherent.

After about an hour and a half I had the worst headache of my life and asked the emergency room Dr. if they could do something about, that I knew from previous experience that it was from the Nitro. The Dr. said unfortunately we need to keep you on the Nitro but he would give me something for the pain.

After about 2 hours or so the came to take me to a Cardiac care center room. The rooms were surprisingly great. They had an atmosphere of home with the walls decorated a 19" color TV with remote and 30 channels of programming. The bed was also something very surprising, it was at first glance an ordinary hospital bed until you got into it and heard the pump kick in. The bed had a self-adjusting air mattress. The mattress would adjust when you move to prevent bed soars and make you more comfortable.

The nurses and aids in the Cardiac Care Unit were fantastic. They were very loving and the most caring hospital nurses I had ever met. They hovered over me like a bunch of mother hens trying to make me as comfortable as possible and showed genuine concern for my condition. At about 8 o'clock that evening I called the nurse in and told her that the headache from the Nitro was unbearable. She said she would call and talk to the Dr.. After about 20 minutes she came back in and removed the small bag of nitro I.V. and put a Nitro patch on my chest. By 10:00 the headache had lessened to a bearable level and I drifted off to sleep.

During the night they checked me several times and at 7:00 the nurses came in and started getting me ready for the heart catheter. At 7:30 the transporter came from the Cath. Lab to take me down to the lab. They wheeled me, bed and all, to the Cath. Lab. Once in the lab the Dr. began to explain what they were going to do. I didn't hear much of what he said, and the next thing I knew, I was back in the room. Seemed like only a few minutes Dr. Grogan came in and said, "We didn't do the Balloon on you Mr. Nigh. I'm thinking, good they didn't find anything. He then said, "Your arteries were to plugged up for the balloon to work, you have 4 completely blocked arteries. That's 4 out of 5 arteries totally blocked.

He said, "Your only chance is to have coronary bypass surgery. I have contacted Dr. Spowart, one of the best cardiac surgeons in California to perform a quadruple by pass tomorrow morning, he'll be in to talk to you shortly and so will the anesthesiologist.

Soon Dr Spowart came in to see me said the usual disclaimer that with any surgery you could die but that chances are I will do fine. He said your going to be operated on at 7:00 AM you should be in recovery in intensive care by noon or so, and later moved to an ICU room until tomorrow when you'll be moved to a Cardiac Care Room. He then asked if I had any questions. I said I couldn't think of any. Soon the Anesthesiologist came in and asked about allergies and if I had ever had a reaction to Anesthesia, I said I hadn't. He also explained what was going to happen and when they would be in to give me a pill and a shot to relax me and they would take me to surgery at around 7:00, once there I would get set up and then be administered the anesthesia.

Very early in the morning, around 5:00 AM the nurses started coming in with medications and soon a beautiful blond nursing assistant came in and said she had to shave me. I said ok and she started to help me take off my gown. I was a little startled, but as she began to shave me she said, they don't want any chance of infection so they have to remove all of my body hair even the armpits and groin area. Soon the transporter came in to take me to surgery. They wheeled me into surgery in the bed from my room just as they had wheeled me to the Cardiac Cath Lab the day before.

When I arrived at surgery I was immediately taken inside and moved to an operating table. The staff in the operating room began to joke with me and I joked back. I noticed that the room was extremely cold and I said, "What is this, a cryogenic chamber to freeze me until medicine has advanced further?" They chuckled and said I would be warm soon, but I haven't been warm since.

Soon I woke up in The Intensive Care Unit about of the hospital in the middle of an open ward with a nurse standing over me saying come on wake up now you've been asleep long enough, you need to wake up now. She was very attractive but had the personality of the nurses in many of the old John Wayne movies. She was a grouch, you know the nurse in the move about Admiral Weed. The one who was a pilot who had to be on crutches for the rest of his life after falling down the stairs at home. So he became a Hollywood writer and was called back to active duty during World War II. He invented the Jeep Carrier. Well, it was about 1:30 in the afternoon I had a tube down my throat so I couldn't answer, but I pointed and nodded to get the tube out of my throat. She said not yet we need to wait.

The tube was gagging me and I felt like I would choke to death if it were not removed immediately. I tried to indicate that to the nurse but she just kept putting me off. I soon became panicked and continued to try to make it clear to her that I needed the tube out of my throat. I kept thinking back to when my dad was dying in the hospital in 1985. He had a breathing tube down his throat and wanted it out so bad that I swear I almost saw him cry. That is how I felt with the breathing tube.

Finally Joan West the surgeons Physicians Assistant came into the ICU to check on me, She was absolutely beautiful, like an angel standing over me. She did some test to see how well I could breath and she then removed the tube from my throat. I immediately began thanking her and she said, you should not talk much right away. I said, OK. She asked me how I felt and I said, "You know that elephant that was sitting on my chest, well he fell through." I had these 2 tubes coming out of my upper abdomen, they were the size of garden hoses, and they were very uncomfortable.

It was very noisy in the ICU ward and about 5:00 the nurse came over to my bed saying there was a big accident and it's going to get very noisy in here soon. We are moving you to an ICU room down at the other end of ICU, you'll have TV. Soon another angelically Beautiful nurse came down and began pushing my bed down to the room at the end of the ward. I was still in the original bed that I started in Thursday afternoon.

The next person to come in to see me was the Physical Therapist, she was also a very beautiful Angel who told me that in the morning she was going to come in and get me started on some workouts. She then said that she was going to help me sit up for a minute and with the help of my nurse got me on my feet, walked me a few steps back and forth then sat me in a chair. I sat there for nearly 15 minutes while she talked to me, then she helped me back to my bed.

Later that evening I began to feel hungry and ask if I could have something to eat. The nurse told me she would check with the Dr. but thought I could only have clear liquids. Soon she came in with a bowl of Jello and said clear liquids was all I could have, but that included Jello. I was so hungry that I eat the Jello too fast and gave myself an upset stomach.

The nurse that came on at midnight was also very beautiful, I'm talking Michelle Pfeiffer Beautiful. The nurse that came on in the morning was a beautiful as well, none however had the special angelic loving personality that the one who took me to that room at 5:00 did. All were very caring and loving however. Soon the lady from dietary came in and asked me what I wanted to eat. She gave me menus to fill out and I filled them out and soon the physical therapist came in got me out of bed and walked me back and forth as far as my chest tubes (the garden hoses) would allow me to go. Then she sat me in the chair.

I sat in the chair for about a half hour until Joan West the PA came in and said she wanted to check to see how the drainage was doing from my chest. She looked and said it looked good and she said I think we can take them out. She had the nurse come in to help, they laid my bed flat, told me that I would feel a little discomfort and to take three deep breaths and she would pull them out on the third breath. One, Two, Three and she pulled. They were out and it felt great.

It was Sunday my wife and son came to see me around noon and stayed for a most of the afternoon. My wife told me that my oldest son Mike and his wife left Saturday morning to come out to see me, but they had car trouble and would be here as soon as they could. The other kids couldn't get away to come out as they had just gotten back to work after being laid off most of the winter. I did talk to the rest of the kids and the grandkids on the phone that day and I was very happy and thankful to be alive.

That evening the nurse said they had a room for me in the Cardiac Care Unit, I would be moving shortly. Ten minutes later Dr. Grogan came in to see how I was doing. In less than a half hour someone came in and said I'm here to take you to CCU. She unplugged my bed and hooked my monitors on a mobile unit and began moving me to CCU.

I arrived in CCU to a bigger room that was very beautiful and so were all the nurses. This hospital had to have the most beautiful and caring nurses in the entire world, you would think I was there father or husband or brother the way they treated me.

In the morning the Nursing Assistant came in to help me get cleaned up and she was like the beautiful sister that you see in the movies all the time who helps her brother to recover from a serious illness by encouraging him and giving him hope. I know that I keep going on about how beautiful all these ladies are, but you would think you hospitalized in a Hollywood made for TV movie or in the show ER. Ever noticed how everyone in the show is beautiful. At Salinas Valley Memorial Hospital that is reality.

Monday morning Joan the PA came in and said that my fluid output was good and was going to remove the catheter, I said great. Soon she had the catheter out and I had more mobility. In a little while the Physical therapist came in and got me out of bed and started walking me around. Soon she said do you feel like taking a little walk, I said sure.

We started out into the hallway and we walked about ten yard and then back to the room where she set me up in the chair. By the time my food tray came I was too tired to continue to set in the chair and eat. I asked to go back to bed to eat. Breakfast stayed down and didn't upset my stomach; I was on the mend.

The next visitor I had was the Dietitian. I was told that I needed to cut my salt down to not more 2000 milligrams per day and to reduce my fat intake to between 30 and 60 milligrams of fat per day. I also need to watch my cholesterol and eat as much cholesterol free foods as possible. I immediately began to try to think of ways that I could follow those dietary restrictions without having to eat that tasteless cardiac diet that they were feeding me in the hospital and that they fed me at The Ft. Hood Hospital 6 years earlier. Later in this book you will find more delicious recipes for a meat and potatoes guy to enjoy and remain on the dietary restrictions that will keep you alive. Those recipes include biscuits and sausage gravy as good as the best you have ever had in any restaurant.

Dr. Grogan came in to see how I was doing he checked my chart and monitors and talked with me for a little while and assured me that in a few days I would be feeling lot better. I said I sure hope so.

My wife's boss Mr. Davis called and asked if I needed anything and I said I could sure use some Caffeine Free Diet Pepsi, so he sent an entire case with my wife. Chaplain Lee and SGM Hendricks called me from USARC Headquarters in Atlanta to see how I was doing. My friend Chuck Clinton called me from Ft McCoy, WI and I received a few cards from the congregation at the Post Chapel.

That evening Dr. Spowart came in and looked at my chart and asked me how I was feeling. I said that I was feeling pretty good considering, he said that I appeared to be recovering nicely.

After several days I began to feel like I was the most loved man in the hospital all of the hospital staff were so loving and friendly they felt like family to me. I wish I could say the same thing about the Chaplain and the headquarters staff at Ft. Hunter Liggett. I hadn't seen anyone from the base yet.

Tuesday afternoon my son and his wife made it to California and to the hospital to see me I was sure happy to see them. They stayed and visited most of the day and that afternoon they went with my wife to get something to eat. After eating they came back and my wife soon left to go home to get my youngest son after school. While they were still there the Installation Commander, LTC Tullar and the Command Sgt. Major came into see me they stayed for only ten or fifteen minutes and then left.

Tuesday evening they moved me to a regular floor, same bed. The staff was not as attentive and a lot more distant. I had a roommate he was a retired military officer but I soon found that he suffered from night terrors. He kept me up until about 2:00 AM when they finally moved him to a room by himself where they could keep the lights on.

I spent that night in the hospital and the next morning Dr. Spowart and Dr. Grogan both came in to see me they both said I was doing well Dr. Grogan said he saw no reason why I couldn't go home this evening. That afternoon they took me to the shower and let me clean up before going home they had me shower with some kind of disinfectant soap like they did when I went in for surgery. My son and his wife picked me up and took me home, my son drove my car and my daughter-in-law drove me in their car.

CHAPTER III

THE RECOVERY

AFTER REACHING HOME I sat down in my recliner as I couldn't go up stairs, but my son had brought down the single bed from our spare bedroom and put it into the dining room and propped up the head in order to make me more comfortable. I quickly learned that propping it up didn't make it very comfortable as I just slid down because it didn't fold in the middle like a hospital bed. If you are going to undergo bypass surgery or any heart surgery you need to make arrangements to get a hospital bed rental and have it delivered to your home before you come home from the hospital. I wound up spending most of my recovery time in the recliner or on the couch, as they were more comfortable.

My son and his wife stayed until Friday morning and left for home as they had to be back to work on Monday. My neighbor and detachment Commander Major Joyner and his wife Jennifer came to see me. They brought the kids Mandy and Brandon because they are like my own grandkids.

I was released with a bunch of prescriptions and the hospital couldn't fill them but they called them into the Rite aid Pharmacy in King City, California. I quickly learned that they didn't have the pain medicine the Dr ordered for me because I am allergic to Morphine, which is the pain drug that is usually prescribed. He prescribed for me Percadan, because I had been prescribed Percadan once when I had chemical burns and it worked and my system tolerated it. I wound up being without pain medicine for 48 hours and I will tell you don't do that. Make sure that you have pain medication when you leave the hospital.

They only stayed for a short time so as not to wear me out. The next morning Chaplain Hartman came to see me and wanted to ask me some questions on how to do something at the Chapel. Later my two assistants and good friends SSG Hamilton and Sgt Darling came to visit me; they were here with the First Battalion 158th Infantry on Operation Noble Eagle to help with Installation security. They brought me a huge canister of black licorice whips, one of my favorite fat free snacks. Their job was to help with spiritual welfare of the soldiers assigned to their unit that included helping with Chapel ministry here at Ft. Hunter Liggett as their headquarters was assigned here.

Shortly after my coming home from the hospital I was asked if I felt like going to the headquarters for my promotion ceremony as I was selected to be promoted effective June 1st, the day I was operated on. LTC Tullar and my wife pinned on my SFC stripes in a formal ceremony at the headquarters building.

Two weeks after the surgery I had a physical scheduled at the U.S. Army Health Clinic at the Presidio of Monterey. I called to see if I should cancel and they said do you feel like coming. I said I did and they said come on in. SGT Darling was my chauffer for the trips to the Dr. both military and civilian. I completed the entire physical by the middle of July and was given a clean bill of health with nothing lower that a 2 on my profile.

As the months passed Jennifer Joyner helped me by taking me to and from the Pharmacy and to the store, as I was unable to drive. I attended church every Sunday starting with the 1st Sunday after getting out of the hospital. Many members of the congregation helped me through this time. Marty and Dave Sizemore really were great.

One Sunday as I was sitting in an easy chair in the back of the sanctuary I was very uncomfortable and Marty said what is wrong. I told that the chair was too hard and she said come sit on the couch. I told her that I would have anyplace to prop my right arm and I couldn't let it hang, it was too hard on my chest. Marty had me come sit by her and prop my right arm on her. You don't know how much that meant to me.

My son Doug and his wife Jamie came with their daughter Taylor the middle of July. When they were here we went to Disney Land and I rented a wheel chair and we enjoyed watching my granddaughter with all the Disney characters and on the rides. While in LA we also went to Hollywood, where we also had and excellent time.

Two weeks after my son Doug and family left we went home for the birth of my grandson Caden who was born the 7th of August to my son Nicholas and his wife Bridget. It was a very exciting time and we enjoyed the visit very much and my Grandson was very cute just like the rest of my grandkids are.

When we returned from Missouri we brought my grandson James, 3 years old with us and planned to meet my daughter in Grand Junction, Colorado over Labor Day weekend since I didn't have to return to work until the Tuesday after Labor Day.

While my grandson was here my son Dustin and I took him and Dustin's friend John Michael camping at Sequoia National Forest. While out there I found that I couldn't breath as good as I could before I had the bypass. We did however have a great time at the park. We saw General Sherman the largest tree in the world and the Crystal Cave.

When we went down to the Crystal Cave it was a mile walk down a steep canyon wall.

There was a spiral path down the canyon wall which took quit a while to walk down but I made it without too much trouble. Then we walked through the cave, which was about a quarter mile walk. Then came the walk back up the canyon wall, this was a very difficult task an took me 3 hours as I could not breath and had to keep stopping to rest.

My grandson, who went camping for the first time in his life, found that he loved camping with Grandpa. The next week I had an appointment with Dr. Grogan's Nurse Practitioner Dawn Tamagni. When I told her that I was having trouble breathing she talked to Dr. Grogan who thought I needed to go to the hospital to have some test run. I was soon admitted to the hospital again to another area of the hospital where I met more beautiful angles of mercy, which took care of me. There was this one nurse from the

Philippines and she was the best she took me for walks and would spend time talking to me. She made me feel like I wasn't alone and that I was with someone who cared.

They ran a chemical stress test after inserting a radioactive dye into my blood and taking a scan of my heart then inserting another chemical into my blood. This chemical put stress on my heart as if I had been running on the treadmill. They monitored me with and EKG while under stress this resulted in a finding that my aortic valve was leaking to badly and if I didn't have it fixed my heart would be worn out in about 10 years.

After I was returned to my room Dr Grogan came in and I had time to think it over and I asked Dr. Grogan if I could wait until after the 1st of October to have the Aortic Valve replacement surgery. He stood there and thought for a moment and said, "Well, you're not in any immediate danger, I don't see any reason why not. You can wait until October it will give you a chance to gain some strength back. I will allow you to return to work on limited duty, no lifting, no mowing, and no strenuous exercise.

I went back to work after taking my grandson to Grand Junction, Colorado to return him to my daughter and son-in-law. On 7 September I returned to work on limited duty. During that time I began setting things up so that I had everything ready for the valve replacement surgery. I got prescriptions set up and got an order for a hospital bed and I closed out the books for the end of the physical year. I opened the new program for my fund and set everything up to have my convalescent leave set up so that I wouldn't have any problems with the Command Sgt Major, CSM Smith. It didn't work. Six days after

I came home from the hospital after my aortic valve replacement I received a Call from The CSM, I'll tell you about that later.

CHAPTER IV

THE AORTIC VALVE REPLACEMENT

On 4 October 2002, as I was preparing to go to the hospital to have my blood work drawn to prepare for surgery on Monday 7 October. Chaplain Hartman came to me and read me a counseling statement for going home while on convalescent leave in August, a leave that he and the Drs all approved. I left the office in discussed and went on to the hospital got my blood work done and went straight to the JAG office. When the JAG opinion came down the counseling statement was thrown out as being frivolous and totally without merit. Needless to say I had a very strenuous weekend.

Sunday night my wife and I went up to Salinas and stayed at the Days Inn because we would have had to get up way to early to be at the hospital on time At 0530 (5:30 AM). 7 October 2002 my wife and I left the motel for the hospital at 0500, I had to be there by 0530 and we made it in good time. Soon they came in with a bag for me to put my clothes in and gave me a gown to put on. In a little while they had my wife leave the room and they shaved my chest, armpits, and groin area again but didn't need to shave my legs this time. The anesthesiologist came in and explained what was about to happen and asked me a few questions. He said, I'll be back. The nursing tech came in and took me down the hall to the shower and had me shower with a special disinfectant soap, in order to avoid infections. Then back to the room to wait for the nurse to give me the pills that will relax me before the anesthesia is administered in the operating room.

A transporter came into the room around 0700 and said we are going to take to surgery now and told my wife she could go to the cafeteria to wait if she liked but that I would probably be in surgery for at least 4-6 hours. My wife went shopping, one of her favorite past times. We started moving down the hallway to surgery, the young transporter and I visiting along the way. Soon we arrived in the Ice Box known as the operating room and I was turned over to the anesthesiologist and soon I was unconscious.

Later that afternoon probably around 1430 or 1500 I woke up and was very uncomfortable. There was a male nurse standing over me and he began asking me how I felt. Was he kidding? I felt like hell, much worse than after the first surgery. He didn't waste a lot of time before he tested to see how I was breathing, my beautiful PA came in and fairly quickly the breathing tube was out. I was still very uncomfortable though because instead of 2, 4 ft garden hoses coming out of my abdomen I had 3 and that felt like something that I can't describe and don't want to. I had a lot of pain that night and took Percadan as often as I could.

In the bed next to me was an older woman who had just had the same thing done that I had and 2 beds down was a guy who also had a valve replacement. He had is breathing tube out also and we began to talk a little, as much as we felt like. The lady still had her breathing tube in and didn't get it out until the next day. On the other side of me was an alcoholic who had been pulled from his car and beaten with ball bats in front of a liqueur store. He was barely alive but was in strong voice. He moaned and groaned for the next 2 days that I was in ICU they didn't have a room in ICU or CCU at the time.

My wife and Chaplain Hartman came into the ICU to see me. Chaplain Hartman didn't stay long but my wife stayed for a few hours. The night went on with lots of moaning and groaning from the old alcoholic. The next morning his daughter who was probably in her late 30s or older and looked like a hippy came in and all day long kept talking to him saying daddy this and daddy that and he kept moaning. If she had used a little common sense and realized that she was in the middle of an ICU ward and talked in a low voice that only her dad could hear it wouldn't have been so bad but she was talking as loud as she could, practically yelling, without actually screaming

Joan the PA came in about 8:00 and checked my chest tubes (the 3 garden hoses) and said we are going to remove them now, just like before I'm going to count to 3 and on 3 I'll pull them out. 1,2,3 and she pulled I thought she was pulling my insides out. Now the biggest portion of the pain was gone. Thank you if I could reach you I would kiss you that feels unbelievable better.

The evening of the second day the lady got her breathing tube out of her throat and she was a very fun lady and very interesting. She had lived a very interesting life but that is another story. The three of us visited and kept each other company. I didn't see the nurses that I had seen in ICU before we seemed to get only male nurses at our end of the ICU, but they were very good and seemed to really care about their patients.

The evening of the 3rd day they finally got me a room in CCU and I moved back to where all the nurses who cared for me the last time were and had not been there very long and the young beautiful nurse from the Philippines came to see me. That made my day and other nurses who had taken care of me before would stop in to see how I was doing.

The next morning I woke up and the nursing assistant came in to help me get cleaned up. She was a gorgeous lady in her late 30s or early 40s and was so loving and helpful. She helped me to the sink so I could shave and I noticed that I had no neck. I looked like and NFL Defensive Lineman or one of those no neck body builders. I said to her this isn't right and she said "No it's not." She got the nurse and about that time My Beautiful PA came in and said I'm going to have Dr. Dox look at you he's in the hall.

Dr. Dox came in and looked and said he was going to send me down to x-ray.

Soon a kid came to take me to x-ray and I took a wheel chair ride. He took several pictures of my chest from different angles, then, sent me back to my room. About a half an hour passed and the x-rays came back and within 20 minutes my room looked like a medical convention. They were bringing in surgical carts, pumps and tubes. Dr. Dox explained to me that he had just come to work for Dr. Spowart to study under one of the best heart surgeons in the country. He told me that he was a Major in the U.S. Army Reserve. He explained that he was getting ready to insert chest tubes as they had nicked both of my lungs when they were removing the adhesions from the 1st surgery. Dr Dox said that my heart looked like someone melted bubble gum and poured it over my heart. They literally had to carve my heart from my chest. The nick in my lungs was causing my chest cavity to fill up with air and would eventually cause my lungs to collapse if they didn't drain the air out of my chest cavity. Dr. Dox Made 2 incisions one on each side of my chest and inserted a long hard plastic straw in each one and secured them to my chest with a single stitch in each one.

After they were done I asked Dr Dox if he would make sure that the proper paper work reached the Presidio of Monterey Medical Clinic for my convalescent leave. He said he would personally make sure that happened.

I spent a week and an half in the hospital. I had a few visitors. About 2 or 3 visits from the Chaplain a couple of visits from my two Chaplain Assistants from the Chapel I had several visits from Major Joiner's wife Jennifer who came up with my wife once and brought her daughter up then brought my son up once. Believe me I was very happy for the visits. Jennifer is like a daughter to me and I don't know how I would have survived this experience without her she was a godsend. Jennifer would take me to my son's football games and take me to the store or run and get things from the store for me. Mandy, Jennifer and Major Joiners daughter would talk to me and help take care of me.

Joann Barber, a nurse who attended our chapel, was a former Army SFC. Joann and her husband served in the Army Medical Corps until she became disabled and he retired. David, her husband, had passed away several years ago. Joann was always Johnny on the spot to give me advise and any help she could. She would take me to COSCO for things we needed that we couldn't get otherwise, and later found ways to help ease my pain. Joann is another person I couldn't have gotten along without.

Just 6 days after I got out of the hospital I received a phone call from CSM Smith, keep in mind that I had not seen nor heard from him or LTC Tullar since I went in the hospital. He began yelling at me saying "SGT Nigh I haven't gotten your paper work for your convalescent leave. Iif I don't have it here by Friday I'm going to file charges against you." I said, "Sgt Major they'll be there, anything else." He said, "Nothing else," and hung up. I called the Presidio and they didn't get the paper work from Dr. Spowart's office yet. I called Dr Spowart's nurse and she told me she would fax the paper work as we spoke. I called the Presidio back and they told me they had them and would do the paperwork for the convalescent leave and fax it today. I thought about what CSM Smith did and thought that LTC Tullar should know what the CSM had said, because it wasn't right. I called the LTC and spoke to him. I explained what had transpired and he said in a rough matter of fact voice "Well if you don't have that paper work in here by Friday I'm going to file something." I said, "Yes sir," and hung up and called the Inspector General's office at USARC. She was appalled, stating that the CSM should have taken care of that himself. This isn't the way a bad soldier should be treated, much less a good soldier with a spotless record. This is not typical for the U.S. Army, most commanders and Sgt Majors are willing to bend over backward to help a soldier who is down in anyway.

I found that my car needed brakes and I couldn't do it myself right now, and it was going to be too expensive for me to have it done in California. Dave Sizemore said he would do it for me. I said fantastic. Now that is what most soldiers are like toward other soldiers who are in need. Dave changed the breaks on the car and wouldn't take any money for doing it. So I gave them some money to buy a gift for their new baby that was due in the spring. I love Dave and Marty like they were my own kids and I hope they know how much I appreciate them and their children who help me not to miss my own grandchildren quite so much.

I received so much support from Katrina and Donald Amos and their daughter Maya while I was convalescing, I couldn't have been more pleased. The members of the Branscome family was very supportive, sending the boys to help my youngest son with things I couldn't do and that Dustin couldn't do by himself. I appreciated them very much.

At Christmas time I talked to my cardiologist about going home for Christmas and there was no problem. My boss the Chaplain had no problem with my going home, but the military Dr., LTC Bussell had other ideas. LTC Bussell stated that I couldn't go home because I needed to stay close to the Surgeon who preformed the surgery in case I would develop complications. Around the 17th of December my family left to go back to Missouri at my insistence to spend Christmas with the rest of the family, I was not going to allow Christmas to be ruined for my grandchildren. When you think about the situation I was alone on a military installation, 80 miles from the Dr and the hospital with most of the soldiers gone home on leave. I have no transportation as was not yet allowed to drive. I have no one at home to check on me in case I become incapacitated. I ask you how is that better for me than traveling to Missouri to be with family where I would be 2 minutes from my old family Dr and 10 minutes from a major hospital with a heart center. Well needless to say, the military Dr wouldn't listen to reason, actually I never even got to talk to him, because he went home for Christmas leave. Well I stayed in my quarters with no car until after Christmas.

I was invited to MAJ Joyner's for Christmas Eve and was asked to spend the night so I could be there when the kids got their Santa presents and opened their other presents in the morning. After the presents were opened and the kids were getting sleepy and ready for naps I went home and called my family to see how Christmas went there. Later that afternoon I went to Donald and Katrina Amos' for another Christmas celebration and to have Christmas supper with them. Several days after Christmas I asked MAJ Joyner to drive me into

King City, 30 Miles away, to get my son's car, which he had left here to sell when he went home after my bypass surgery. I now had wheels.

My wife and son returned on 5 January and on 7 January I had a Dr appointment to get my clearance to return to work. I was told that I would have to have a Medical Evaluation Board to determine if I could stay in the Army, or if I would be forced to retire on disability. The prospect at this point in my life of retirement was not what I wanted to do. I was still young and vital, although when I was about 25 I thought I would retire at age 50 and travel the world, but at age 53 the reality of economics had set in and the reality of inflation. I was not a happy camper. As the days went on so did the medical appointments, the constant probing and sticking me every week for blood.

The more I thought about it the better playing with my grandkids the rest of my life sounded. I still was worried about the financial end of the whole thing. The pressures here in the Army and the harassment from those in authority who don't like it when a soldier got to retire before them got to be too much and in March of 2003 I had an angina attack. I got really week, my chest started hurting and I got dizzy. I was at work on Sunday morning and I called 911 and the ambulance came. The Paramedics checked my blood pressure and could only get a top reading which was 50 by palp. I was rushed to the hospital and after three days I was told that it was stress related and that I would be ok but I should take the rest of the week off. I received a week's convalescent leave and a month later was told to quit working 6 days a week.

Well naturally the Army couldn't leave that alone the military Dr put on my permanent profile that I was not to work over 40 hours per week. Well the Chaplain decided that if he didn't count my breaks and my Physical Training time or any of the extra duties I do that I could still work 6 days a week, event-though I would not be excused from any of the above. So I began keeping a log of the hours I was asked to work to accomplish the jobs I was assigned to do and I since turning the record over to the Dr. I started getting off, due to reaching my 40 hours, around noon on Thursdays.

I love my job as a Chaplain Assistant because I get to be a soldier and serve God and my Country at the same time. I can think of no more rewarding career for a dedicated young Christian to be involved in. I had my Medical Evaluation Board on 3 June 2003 and I appealed it. I had my PEB on 12 June 2003 and appealed it because they only gave me 30% when the guidelines they sent state that more than one (1) episode of congestive heart failure in 1 year resulting in hospitalization is a minimum of 60%, heck I had 4 hospitalizations for heart related failure in 9 months. 18 June I appeared in front of the Physical Evaluation Board appeal committee. The JAG lawyer stated that I should get the 60% without to much problem. The Army Medical Board in their infinite wisdom chose to give me only 30%, I appealed the decision based on the Army's own guidelines that stated more than one episode of congestive heart failure within one year constitutes 100% disability I had 2 within 4 months. The Army on appeal still only gave me 30%. I applied for V.A. disability, eventually receiving 100%. If the Army had given me 100% they would have had to pay me 75% of my base pay on concurrent receipt which means my full 75% Army retirement along with my V.A. disability. Currently they are offsetting my retirement to pay to the V.A. until I reach age 60.

CHAPTER V

LIVING WITH HEART DISEASE

HEAR IS WHERE WE get into the real nitty-gritty, this chapter will tell you how to deal with the disease and improve your life style while helping to prevent future heart attacks and open heart surgery through Diet, exercise and proper medication. I will also give you list of alternative over the counter and experimental programs that will give you some insight into contacting people who can help you prevent the incurrence of the problems I have had, by cleaning out your arteries before they get to the point that you need surgery. I will make references to my own diet that has been reviewed and approved by Cardiologists, Dietitians, Physical Therapists and Home Health Nurses. I will also refer you to information that was given to me by Salinas Valley Memorial Hospital and by the Monterey County Visiting Nurse Service.

Once the surgeons have cracked your chest, when you awake you will be given a heart shaped pillow and told that this is your lifeline. When you get up, cough, sneeze or just change positions you will need to hug this pillow to protect your chest and it helps reduce the pain level from moving. When you get out of the hospital and are no longer taking pain medication you will find that your cloths will irritate your chest and your incision, mainly your left chest where they removed the mammary artery. If you will take a piece of saran wrap or other plastic wrap and place on your chest before you get dressed you will notice that you are much more comfortable and are not always tugging at your shirt. If you find that the plastic wrap doesn't stay in place, well try putting a little hand lotion on the area before putting the plastic wrap on. As a last resort use a couple of small pieces of tape to hold it in place. Dr. Grogan's nurse Kimmie gave this little tidbit to me. If you can get your Dr. to write you a prescription Lidoderm patches they are wonderful, you can cut them in half and place on either side of your scar until it is healed enough then place it over the whole thing.

The Respiratory Therapist will give you a little contraption that you can suck air from that measures how your lungs are expanding and will help you to expand them so that you get your breathing back to normal and don't develop pneumonia. You need to use this device as often as the Therapist tells you to. Try to get to the top as soon as you can and draw your breath slowly, which will expand your lungs much more quickly.

Soon when you are able to eat they will bring you a bunch of food to eat that is not seasoned with any salt and is very low fat. They will tell you that if you want to survive you will need to change your eating habits and begin eating more like the diet that you are provided in the hospital. Well the come back to that is that they are right but you don't have to give up all the foods that you love nor do you have to give up taste. You will simply need to learn to prepare your foods differently than you have in the past.

PAM cooking spray and olive oil will soon become your best friends in the kitchen.

I have learned to eat around 30 grams of fat per day and on occasion I will go to 60 grams of fat per day. 60 grams of fat is what the

USDA, the AMA and the American Heart Association agree is the daily amount of fat that an average healthy person should eat, however the average American eats between 150 and 300 grams of fat per day. 25 to 50 times more than we should. With places like McDonalds, who won't even serve a ranch dressing for their side salad that has less that 30 grams of fat unless you like French or Italian. That right the Newman's Own Ranch salad dressing that McDonalds serves has 30 grams of fat per serving. About the only thing that is on McDonalds menu that you can eat on a 30 gram of fat a day diet is their breakfast burrito and they don't have that at every McDonalds. Here in California you can get a Chorizo Burrito that is not healthy as it is loaded with fat and 3 times the size of a McDonalds Breakfast Burrito.

About 6 weeks after surgery you will need to start exercising. Start out slowly and walk on the treadmill at about 2 to 2.5 miles per hour for about 10 minutes making sure that you do not exceed the maximum heart rate that your Dr has set out for you. Do that for about a week and then go for 14 minutes keeping track of heart rate and not exceed the limit set by your Dr.. The 3rd week you can go up to about 17 minutes, and on the 4th week you can go up to 20 minutes, now at each of these levels. If you see that you are having trouble you need to cut back to a level that doesn't stress you too much and doesn't exceed the maximum heart rate that your Dr has set for you. Once you have reached the 20-minute level and had no problems maintaining your speed for 20 minutes for an entire week its time to speed up. Go to 2.8 miles an hour for a couple of days and see how you feel, if you have no problems go to 3 miles per hour. Then after going 3 miles per hour for 20 minutes for one week you can then speed up to 3.5 miles per hour your goal is to reach 4.3 miles per hour for 35 minutes by increasing a little each week until you reach that level. You must realize that these numbers are for someone who was physically fit before have the open heart surgery, and I know that sounds like some type of Oxymoron but being in shape is the only reason that I didn't have a massive heart attack and die. If you were not in shape before the surgery now is the time to get into shape.

You need to start slower maybe at 1.5 miles per hour for 10 minutes. You need to get to that 20 minute mark as soon as you possible can. Continue from there with speed increases until you reach at least 4.0 miles per hour then start increasing your times until you can get to 35 minutes. I feel that 4 miles per hour for at least 35 minutes will be the magic number for you to shoot for and for you to maintain your fitness in the future. While you are recovering you should do this every weekday taking the weekends off to rest. Once in shape you can cut back to 3 days per week, Monday, Wednesday and Friday are great.

Now we need to look at some ways of preventing you from having to go through the agony of open-heart surgery by clearing your arteries of plaque before you need to have a bypass.

The first thing we are going to talk about is proper diet has much to contribute to heart disease prevention. With prevention in mind, your diet should be rich in vitamins, minerals, and other nutrients that combat high blood pressure, excessive clot formation, and arteriosclerosis. Particularly noteworthy clot reducing nutrients include potassium, magnesium, vitamin E and the essential fatty acids contained in fish oils. Some studies suggest that selenium may also protect against heart disease and stroke. A low-fat diet loaded with fruits and vegetables, however, is probably the best nutrition-related preventive step you can take for both heart attack and stroke.

Probably raising the antioxidant levels in the blood is the single most important step you can take to prevent heart attack or stroke.

Doctors have been telling people for years to eat more fruits and vegetables but have not been stressing it enough as they seem to be more concerned with your cholesterol and blood pressure. The truth is according to a study by the World Health Organization the antioxidant status is actually more important.

According to the study, which studied thousands of men and women from 16 nations, low levels of vitamin E in the blood are better than twice the predictor of heart attack than cholesterol or high blood pressure. Research conducted by the Rockefeller University shows that supplementation with N-acetyl-cysteine (NAC) lowered blood levels of the most dangerous cholesterol fraction, Known as lipoprotein (a), by 70 percent. Research that was published in the American Journal of Clinical Nutrition states that blood levels of vitamin C are inversely related to blood pressure. As vitamin C levels increase in the blood that blood pressure decreases. There is a good book by Stephen Cherniske, M.S., "The Metabolic Plan Stay Younger Longer" that explains more about this and how

DHEA and restoring your anabolic metabolism will dramatically reduce your risk of cardiovascular disease. His book talks about these studies and others published in the New England Journal of Medicine and the Journal of Clinical Endocrinology and Metabolism.

An Article written by Dr. Robert Jay Rowen's titled "Building Super Immunity by Feeding Your Body Extra Oxygen". It states that Cancer, high blood pressure, obesity, arthritis, heart disease, colds and flu, depression, strokes and over 100 other life-threatening problems can be delayed, prevented or reversed by giving your body the extra oxygen it's craving. You can live a longer, healthier, more energetic life at any age.

The first therapy he talks about is hyperbaric oxygen therapy. Next he talks about ozone therapy. Last he talks about EWOT (exercise with oxygen therapy) all seem to be very sound principles and bare checking into in order to help you stay healthy or to get healthier.

There are many different therapies and theories that will help you to prevent a heart attack or stroke. In addition to the therapies described below, you might want to consult a practitioner of Chinese medicine or a homeopathic physician for treatment of post-heart surgery or stroke complications. Acupuncture, for example, is endorsed by the World Health Organization as a viable stroke rehabilitation therapy. This will alleviate the pain following open-heart surgery. Make sure that you clear this with your cardiologist or physician as these treatments and medications my have negative effects on the medications prescribed by your Dr.. One of these potential homeopathic medications is Vitalzyme. It's an enzyme that is said to remove plaque from the blood stream and to turn scar tissue back into healthy normal tissue. At present my cardiologist is looking into the effects of this enzyme as it is said to eliminate the need to do further surgery on patients to remove post surgical adhesions as well as eliminating plaque from the blood.

If, like myself you have had a valve replacement with a metal valve the use of this product must be monitored very closely by a physician as it is also a blood thinner and can have a serious negative effect when you are taking cumadin.

If your risk of heart attack is high due to family history or stroke is high because of severe arteriosclerosis, high blood pressure, or a history of heart disease, TIAs, or previous strokes, you should see a doctor regularly. If the indicated danger is clot stroke, your doctor may advise a baby aspirin (81mg) a day to thin your blood. If you have diabetes, control it, since it increases your risk of stroke.

There are Herbal Therapies: A number of scientific studies have shown that Ginkgo biloba (ginkgo increases cerebral blood flow, so it may be helpful in moderating potential complications of stroke such as disturbed thought processes, memory loss, symptoms of depression and vertigo. Ginkgo also appears to reduce instances of blood-clot formation, which will help reduce the chances of a heart attack and stroke. Many other herbs are said to be useful in heart attack and stroke prevention because of their abilities to improve circulation, reduce clot formation, strengthen and tone blood vessels, and combat arteriosclerosis, but as always consult your physician before taking any over the counter medications.

Several bodywork techniques can help restore mobility, promote circulation, and ease muscle tension and stiffness associated with open-heart surgery and stroke. Among these are qigong, shiatsu, and massage, and electro therapy, which restore your body's electrical energy and help it to focus that energy toward repairing damage or illness but check with your Dr before beginning any type of alternative therapy.

Techniques that teach the body to relax and the mind to focus on healing can help recovering heart attack and stroke victims; among other benefits, these techniques can increase tolerance to pain and also alleviate the anger or depression that is common after major surgery or stroke. Meditation, hypnotherapy and yoga all can be useful to some heart attack victims working to restore lost muscle tone from biofeedback.

Chiropractic and Osteopathy: These two closely related manipulative therapies could aid heart surgery recovery in numerous ways. By focusing on realignment of the body's skeletal system, they may be able to reduce muscle spasms and stiffness, improve mobility, alleviate nagging pains, and minimize further stress due to spinal misalignment allowing your body to focus on the healing process of the heart.

Measures that reduce the chances of heart attack or stroke are: Adopt habits that promote cardiovascular health and deter arteriosclerosis. The essentials of a healthy lifestyle include eating foods that are low in fat, salt, and cholesterol; exercising regularly; controlling weight; monitoring blood pressure and cholesterol levels; limiting alcohol; and not smoking.

You or someone around you has manifest any of the signs of heart attack including chest pains, numbness or tingling in the left arm or difficulty breathing, these are symptoms of heart attack. If the symptoms pass quickly, this may indicate angina, this is a period of extreme stress on the heart that is usually a forerunner to heart attack. If someone experiences the symptoms of stroke and the symptoms pass quickly this may be a transient ischemic attack (TIA), this is often a forerunner to stroke it is a brief blockage of blood flow to the brain. Do not ignore these signs; immediate medical attention is essential.

I. V. kelation therapy is another route that you can look into if you are at risk for heart disease or stroke. This is a method that was devised to remove heavy metals from the blood, for example people with prolonged lead exposure. The Drs who began using this technique have discovered that it also reduces the amount of plaque in the blood (plaque being the primary cause of arterial blockage). The American Medical Association has not yet made a decision on weather or not the process actually reduces the chance of heart attack nor has the American Heart Association and they are still studying the matter but a number of heart surgeons believe this is the only way to go. Dr Isadore Rosenfeld of

Wild Cornell University said on his program on Fox news channel, "There is no evidence that this procedure is in anyway harmful and there is evidence that it does work in removing heavy metal. So for people who are at risk for potential heart disease it couldn't hurt, talk to your Dr."

The main thing that you need to remember is if you have chest pain and it is so sever that you believe you're having a heart attack take an aspirin and see your Doctor or get to the emergency room as quickly as possible, your live may depend on it.

Now I am going to give you the most important advice in this book. If the doctors try to pass it off as nothing get a second opinion and third opinion if necessary, because you know your body better than anyone else, and the quicker you can get your heart problems fixed the less invasive the procedures will be. Hypochondriacs live conger than most other people because their medical problems are usually caught in the early treatable stages. If caught early enough you can get by with the non invasive procedures that I just talked about, or at worst a heart cath with balloons and stints.

If you are put off or wait to long like me, you will wind up having to have bypass surgery. That in its self is bad enough, but make sure that your doctors discuss every aspect of your pending surgery with you, I did not, that is why I had to be opened up a second time four months after my by pass. I am now suffering from Acute Pain Syndrome which happens to one in three thousand open heart surgery patients. Acute Pain Syndrome is a condition that happens when the nerves are severed and continue firing and telling your brain that you are in pain. Most people who experience this condition suffer low levels of pain constantly, on a pain scale of 1-10, ten being the worst pain you have ever experienced, people with Acute Pain Syndrome experience pain levels of less than 5 mostly around 2 or 3. Some people 1 in 1,000,000 experience pain of more than 5, in my case without pain medication my pain levels are 9 or 10. even with medication my pain levels are never below 5 until the pain Drs. put me on Lyrica a drug developed for Rumatoid Arthritis but was found to help people with Fibermoraldia which is a disease of the nerves and has helped me to get off the narcotic pain medications.

When you experience pain levels of 2-5 on a constant basis you will suffer as the longer the pain is there the more it wears on you and the worse you feel. When your pain levels are in excess of 5 on a daily basis, even when you have been taught to overlook pain as I have, you will eventually get to the point where you will be praying for God to take you home. Especially when the doctors tell you that they can't do anything to help except give you narcotic drugs on a daily basis. Don't give up because if you do you will loose hope and with out hope you will most likely loose your will to live, and without that hope you will surely die.

I have been to the Neurology Clinic at Kansas University Medical Center in

Kansas City, Kansas and have been given neuron ton which didn't work. I was also given a set of electrodes and a battery operated power supply to stimulate the muscles and nerves to try to relieve the pain. It worked to a degree while I was hooked up to the machine but as soon is I shut if off the pain returned. In 2005 I was given a pace maker because my heart wouldn't speed up during exercise and could no longer use the electrodes. I have been given several different types of Anti Depressants and nerve medications. None worked.

I went to the head of thoracic Surgery at St. Luke's Hospital in Kansas City,

Missouri and had he wires removed from my chest and checked to make sure that there is no movement of my sternum. The sternum was solid and removing the wires helped the pain a little bit for a short time.

I have been to the Pain Canter at Heartland Regional Medical Center in St.

Joseph, Missouri, and Dr. Beattie, who I respect very much has tried trigger point injections, they didn't work, He stated that I would need to be on drugs for the pain for ever that he didn't know any thing else to do short of putting in a Dilated pump, Morphine is the usual choice but I'm allergic to Morphine. I don't at this point want to settle for just masking the pain and loosing my self.

I went to go to the pain center at Kansas University Medical Center. and If that didn't yield results then I was prepared go the Pain Center at Mayo Clinic in Rochester, Minnesota The main thing is that I haven't given up and I am still here. The Drs. at the pain center at Kansas University Medical Center pain clinic prescribed for me the Lyrica described above and the results where that they lowered my pain levels to where without narcotics on the 1-10 scale were at 4.

The most important thing to remember when you have heart disease is never take anything for granted, such as a moderate chest pain or shortness of breath. I have been short of breath for the past 5 years and it has been steadily getting worse. I have been telling my cardiologists about the pain and shortness of breath and in the last five years I have received a total of 5 stints and a pace maker. 6 weeks ago I was diagnosed with an enlarged Aorta, I was told also that I needed to have it replaced. Because I have to be on Plavix and Aspirin for the rest of my life because of the stints that if I want to continue to do things like ride horses the neurologists said that I needed to get off cumadin. The only way to get off cumadin is to replace the metal valve with a tissue valve. I was told that I also needed another bypass and need to have my pacemaker replaced so that it won't shock me like it did in April. This is information for the next chapter.

CHAPTER VI

ANOTHER OPEN HEART SURGERY

Since I retired I tried to return to work with the Missouri Department of Corrections in December of 2003 the week of Christmas, I worked 3 days that week and 3 days the week of New Years, then 1 1/2 Days after New Years. I went to the Dr. on Tuesday afternoon and was diagnosed with congestive heart failure. I was Immediately sent to the hospital at St. Johns in Leavenworth, Kansas where I spent the next month. While there I had several test run. In one of the test I was administered the wrong radioactive die, because the two technicians were to busy constantly arguing with each other to pay attention. In April of 2003 I had a Heart Catheterization at Providence Hospital in Kansas City, Kansas.

I went to the hospital and it took 3 nurses 5 sticks to get an IV started in my very large and visible veins, soon I was wheeled into the cath room the nurses where very nice, attractive ladies who seemed to be very knowledgeable and dedicated to their jobs. During the Cath Dr. Masrani ordered extra contrasting die. The die was administered, I was watching the whole thing, the next thing I knew I had a nurse sitting on my chest yelling breath, so I took a gasping breath, she then said now cough, I coughed she then stated he's back.

I later found out that my heart had stopped due to getting too much die. I died for a short time, I guess I wasn't gone long enough to have an out of body experience. They then sent me back to my room without doing anything else that day. Dr. Masrani then had me come back the Wednesday before Memorial Day when they did another heart cath, a balloon angioplasty and a stint placement, the first of 5. After I was sent to my room the nurse checked my cath site and found that it was bleeding. The nurse held pressure on the wound site and maintained that pressure for about 6 hours then a plastic knob and a sand bag were placed at the cath site and I had to sleep flat on my back until morning.

On Saturday I was released to go home. My family had planned a trip to the Henry Doorley Zoo in Omaha, Nebraska, so when they picked me up we took off even though I was black and blue and soar from my knees to my nipples. We had a great time even though my sons had to push me through the zoo in a giant stroller.

In July I went into Provident Hospital and received 2 more balloons and stints, I again had to be stuck at least 3 or 4 times before they could get the I.V. started. I don't remember much about this cath except that It was uneventful except for the placement of the 2nd and 3rd stint. Again the nurses were fantastic I didn't like having to lay flat for the first 8 hours as it made my back hurt.

In August I Shawnee Mission medical center for my 4th stint and this time it took only one stick to get the I.V. in. I have never had a problem having I.V.s put in before or since. I don't remember anything about that stint placement or even the cath because they again knocked me out. I do remember the wonderful nurses and the great post procedure care I received.

I n April of 2005 I had a stress test at which time I was told that my heart was not speeding up and that I needed a pacemaker to help my heart speed up when I exerted during physical exercise. On 5 May 2005 I received a Guidant Pacemaker at the Cushing Hospital in Leavenworth, Kansas as an out patient procedure, after that procedure I was able to breath well enough that I could walk all over the 36 acre ranch that I had just bought.

On 15 May 2005 we started construction of our new house. In June I had chest pains at the construction site and called an ambulance and was taken to Heartland Hospital in St. Joseph, Missouri. I was there for 4 days and had several test and was told that I had an angina attack. In November we moved into our new house just before Thanksgiving. In 2006 I began having shortness of breath again and was told that I should just cut back on my activities in in October of 2006 I changed cardiologist to Drs. Kevin Muller and David Wiley at Mid American Cardiology at K. U. Medical Center.

In January I felt so bad, weak, short of breath and tired all the time that when my wife and kids decided to take me to this really nice restaurant in Kansas City. I really didn't feel like going but I went. We left at 12:30PM and I rode to the restaurant approximately an hour waited 2 hours for a table and another hour and a half to be waited on and get our food. On the way home at around 6:00 PM I was told that we were going to my brothers house for ice cream and cake. I said I can't do it I need to go home and my wife said that we planned this nice birthday for you and all you want to do is go home. All you ever do is think about yourself. I said that I didn't think that they even thought about me when they planned the birthday or they wouldn't have drug me allover knowing how bad I felt.

I then said let's go to my brothers. At 8:00 PM I had one of my kids take me home.

In February of 2007 I was taken to the hospital by ambulance to Heartland Hospital in St. Joseph, Missouri where I told them that I didn't want Dr. Lamoglia anywhere near me or even in the same room with me. For 3 days they kept trying to push me to let Dr. Lamoglia do the heart cath they finally had Dr. Hindapur do it and he said their was no blockage and he was going to give me 7 mg of cumadin and send me home the next day. I said no you are not going to give me 7 mg of cumadin because my INR would reach 8.5 by morning as it did when the first placed my aortic valve and gave me 7 mg. He then sent the nurse in with a 5 mg tablet and said I could take 5 mg and go home in the morning. I told the nurse that my INR would probably be high when I had I checked in 2 days. I took it because I needed to get away from these two inept Doctors, when I had my INR checked it was 5.4 nearly double what it was suppose to be. I went home and my breathing continued to get worse and I continued to get weaker by the day.

After 3 weeks I called my Cardiologist's office and told the nurse how bad I felt and she talked to the Dr. who said that I needed to have a stress echo. The nurse told me that the Dr. wanted to do the stress echo at K.U.. and it would be another 3 weeks before they could get me in. I said that was fine and on March 29th 2007 I drove to K.U.. Medical Center and walked into the cath lab area where the stress echo was to be administered

The technician said that I looked gray and they didn't want me to have a heart attack on the bicycle during the test so she was going to do an echo to see what she could see. She began the echo and soon printed off a few pages and said I'll be right back. I need to talk to the

Dr., She and the Dr. returned in a few minutes. The Dr. said that they were going to admit me to the cath lab and do a cath the next day something just didn't look right.

The next morning I was prepped for the cath and at noon was taken to the cath lab and by the way they hit my veins the first try. When I came out of the lab I was told that I they found a 85% blockage in one of my main arteries so they stinted it with a bear metal stint, because of the 4 sifer drug alluding stints which have been plugging up since the were put in.

In April I was watching TV and talking on the Telephone when my pacemaker shorted out and shocked me in the left shoulder so severely that it paralyzed my left arm for 12 hours. I was in severe pain that entire time. I was taken to Heartland Hospital and admitted I told them upon admission that I wanted to be transferred to K.U ... Medical Center. It was the next afternoon before they transferred me to K.U ... I was told that my pacemaker was now working but there was no data for the 12 hour period that my arm was paralyzed and that I was in extreme pain.

In May I had chest pains again and was again taken to Heartland Hospital by ambulance and was immediately transferred to K.U.. where I spent about a week before being sent home with the Drs. Telling me that I had had a minor heart attack. They tried to tweak my pacemaker and said come see Dr. Wiley on July 19th because Dr Mulhern would be on vacation at that time. On July 19th I was again hospitalized for a week at

K. U. Medical Center. During the month of August I had several test run and was in and out of the Drs. Offices 2 and 3 times a week.

On September 3rd I saddled up my horse and went for a ride, we had a good ride and were heading back to the barn on a run when

Princess stumbled on an uneven piece of ground. My synch slipped and my saddle slipped sideways. I hit the ground on my back and my head never even came close to the ground, as a matter of fact my cowboy hat never left my head. The wind wasn't even knocked out of me and Princess stopped came back and bent down so that I could grab her halter and she helped me up. She and I walked back the 15 yards to the barn where I unsaddled her and my brother and I went in the house to watch TV. About 4 hours latter I had a headache so bad that I couldn't stand it my brother told me I better call the Dr. because I could have had a clot break loose and go to my brain.

After talking to the on call Dr. at Mid American Cardiology, who told me that he didn't think that it was heart related but that he strongly, strongly, strongly suggested that I go the Emergency room at St. Luke's North, so my brother took me. As soon as we walked in the door I was taken into a room no waiting in the waiting room for an hour and within 5 minute I was in CAT scan and then back to the room. It didn't seem like 5 maybe 10 minutes and the Dr. was in my room stating that I had a Subdural Hematoma and need to be transferred to a trauma center. I asked if I could be sent to K.U.. Medical Center. The Dr. said that they would check. He returned to the room saying that K.U.. Medical Center E.R.. was closed, which meant that K.U.. was more than 80% full and some of the other hospitals in K.C.. weren't and he explained that St. Luke's has some of the best trauma and neurologist in North West Missouri so I went to St. Luke's.

On Wednesday September 5th I woke up blind, I could only see light and movement, the Drs. Said that the blood was pooling in my occipital lobe was way I couldn't see. I ask how long before it would clear up? He said that it might never clear up and that was a very likely prospect. The prospect of being blind for the rest of my life was one thing that really terrified me. The next day I woke up and my sight was returning I could see in the center but was still blurry and unable to focus around the outer edges. As usual I beat the odds and was getting better despite what the Drs said. After nearly 3 month might sight never went back to as clear as it was before.

I spent 1 week in neurological ICU and one week the stroke ward before being sent home on Saturday September 15th on Monday the 17th I had chest pains and called the Mid American Cardiology and was instructed to go to the emergency room. I called the ambulance and they came and checked me out and said that I need to go to the emergency room but they couldn't take me to K.U.. so I said forget it. I then called my wife and she and my daughter came and picked me up and took me to K.U.. where I stayed for the next 2 weeks returning home on the 29th of September.

While in the hospital I had a mini stroke on the 3rd day and I was told that I should be off cumadin for the rest of my life. The risk for stroke from being on cumadin, plavix and aspirin, a deadly combination but because of the mini stroke which was from a clot that broke loose from my heart valve. I was placed on 1 mg of cumadin per day them wanting my INR at about 1.5-2.0. It was decided that I would return to Dr. Gorton's office on 29 October to set the date for my surgery to remove my metal aortic valve and replace my aorta and with a bovine valve which needs no additional medication. Yea! No more cumadin. At the same time Dr. Gorton would also do a by-pass and while I am in the hospital they would also replace my pacemaker. Whoa! No more waiting for the other shoe to drop, and this time it could kill me if it shorts out again.

Well Dr. Gorton and I decided that I would go into the hospital after stopping my cumadin after my Friday dose on Tuesday 6 November and would have the surgery tentatively on Thursday 8 November if my blood work looks good.

November 6th my wife and sister-in-law took me to K.U.. we arrived at about 9:30 AM. I checked in at the desk of the Heart Center and was instructed to have a seat in the waiting area. The three of us sat down in some very comfortable chairs and waited, but we saw a coffee shop and I got a iced mocha blended coffee that was absolutely delicious.

After about 15-20 minutes an admitting clerk called me, we filled out the paper work and I was asked to wait back in the waiting 5-10 minutes for a transporter. In about that amount of time a really nice looking sweat young lady came to take me to my room which was Cardio Thoracic Surgery Progressive Care Unit room 11, CTS PCU 11 where I was met by a beautiful Nurse named Allison and a beautiful Nursing Tech named Amy they were wonderful and were Johnny-on-the-spot all day long making sure that I was comfortable and well cared for. One of the Drs. Came in to see me and discussed a little about the surgery and stated that I would most likely be on the top of the surgery schedule for Thursday the 8th.

On Tuesday evening I got a new nurse and tech, they were also gorgeous, their names were, Nurse Liz and the tech was Mikea my nurse gave me extremely close care and was on top of my Heparin IV all night because my Heparin levels kept getting to high.

Wednesday morning at 7:00 am shift changed again and my nurse was a pretty girl named Erin and my tech was a lovely girl named Lois the care they gave me was the best in the world.

Thursday morning around 5:00 AM or 0500 for you military types the nurses came and told me that they would be taking me at around 8:00 AM for surgery. Around 6:00 AM the nurse came in and said you need to take your second disinfecting shower. They thought I would need my acid reflux medicine and my Coreg. At around 7:00 my Wife, Daughter, Sister-in-law, and my brother Albert came to give me support. At shortly after 8:00 AM the transporter from surgery came to my room transferred me to a gurney and headed for surgery.

Once I arrived at surgical floor I was shaved all over my body and given something to relax me. Soon they were putting in an arterial line in my right arm as well as a second I.V.. Shortly after that they put in the arterial line in my neck I was pretty well out of it when they put in the line in my neck.

The next thing I know I'm waking up in I.C.U. with that dreaded breathing tube down my throat and I motioned for the nurse to take it out. She said you have had a really bad time and it's 12:30 A.M. Friday we need to make sure that you are ok and don't have to go back to surgery before we take it out. She said you bled so severely that you had to be given quit a bit of blood products. They finally took out the tube around 2:40 A.M. and they watched me very closely until about 8:40 A.M. they brought me a liquid breakfast.

The breakfast tasted really good, it consisted of some kid of fruit juice mixture.

About 11:30 I was transferred from I.C.U. to the Post Cardiac Surgery floor which was the third floor of the cardiac wing. I had the same nurses that I had before I had surgery.

Around noon I got a light lunch and by supper time I was eating a normal cardiac diet.

I was surprisingly in much less pain than I expected, probably because I had been in so much pain for so long that I had grown use to it. Friday night my pain levels did not allowed me to sleep and by Saturday morning we had them down. Sunday morning my pain levels came back up because I didn't get the pain meds on schedule. By

Kick-off time of the Kansas City Chiefs game my pain was back under control, so much so that I wore my Tony Gonzalez Jersey number 88 it was an exciting game even though we lost, but still retain the lead in the AFC WEST. I have been a Chiefs fan since they came from Dallas in 1960 and changed their name from the Dallas Texans to the Kansas City Chiefs.

My wife, daughter, brother Albert, sister-in-law Mary and 3 of my grandkids came to see me. I love to have visitors in the hospital. We had a great visit and I was surprised at how well I felt all day.

Sunday morning I was really in a lot of pain and thought it was because of all of the commotion that I had Saturday. At 10:00 A.M. the P.A. from Dr. Gorton's office came in and said are you ready to get those chest tubes out. He took off the tape and loosened the stitches then counted to three, I took a deep breath and he pulled them out. By noon we had my pain pretty much at a manageable level.

Monday morning I woke up and I could feel the pain coming on strong and asked for my pain meds and the tech said that my nurse was giving report and it could be a while.

By the time the nurse came in my pain level had grown to a ten and it took all day to get it under control. I talked to the Dr. when he came in and requested that they wake me up in the night to give me the pain meds on schedule. He issued an order for them to wake me to give me the pain meds. The thing that you need to remember is not that if you are sleeping that your pain must be under control. What you need to remember is if you don't stay on schedule that when you wake up that your pain could be out of control before you get the meds. At around 10:A.M. the nurse removed my Foley catheter.

Tuesday morning 9:00 Dr. Gorton came in and said are you ready to go home. I said that my pain was under control, that I was eating regularly, urinating ok and my bowels were moving without discomfort, so yeah. Ok, he said, I'll sign your release and we'll get you out of here. I called my wife and she said it could be a while before she could get down, I said no hurry. About 10:15 A.M. my son Nick called me and said he had just passed Dearborn, MO. and he was on the way to get me and asked me how long did I think it would be before he would get to K.U.., I said probably 40 minutes. Nick said he had concrete coming to pour his front porch at 3:00 P.M.. I said, no worries, I'm dressed and ready, I just need to get my last I.V. out. He got there at around 11:15 and by 12:20 we were in out way. We stopped at Ft. Leavenworth to pickup my prescriptions.

We arrived home at around 2:45 and Nick headed next door to his house to wait for the concrete truck. Now I face about 6 weeks recovery time, but this time I know that as soon as they replace my defective pacemaker in about 3 weeks I will feeling better than I have for years.

After going home I went to the pacemaker Dr. who stated that my heart was now pacing up to 135 beats per minute. He then said I really didn't need the pacemaker anymore but he didn't know how it could have caused the shock that I felt in April, it's only 9 volts. I didn't think of it at the time but did you ever put a brand new fully charged 9 volt battery on your tongue, imagine that then think about that kind of shock on bare tissue. The Dr. then stated that he wouldn't take it out because it could cause the leads to tear the heart and then they would have to open me back up and I could die before they could get in.

On 8 December 2007 we had an unbelievable ice storm. It knocked out power to thousands of people in Northwest Missouri. I was feeling so good, and I am the Chaplain for the Disaster Relief Chain Saw Team from our church so I went out with the team and helped drag brush to the curb for 2 weeks. I only worked about 2 hours then we took an hour and a half lunch then I worked another hour then went home. Then Christmas I felt a little punk but I managed to keep going around the house until New Years Eve when I went out to feed the horses, came back in and started to unload the dishwasher when I started shivering and at the same time was burning up. I called my wife and told her I need to go the K.U.. Medical Center I knew why I was feeling so bad for the past week, my malaria was back. She came home and took me to the hospital where they ran blood test and found it wasn't malaria but I had a temperature of 104.9 and for an mature adult that is a drastically high temperature. After a week in the hospital I went home feeling very little better but had no temperature. The Drs. Said that I had gotten a viral infection that had gone to my heart but didn't do any permanent damage and it would take about 4-6 weeks before I felt better. Bottom line here is no matter how good you feel after open heart surgery you need to remember is you are very fragile and your immune system is taxed to the max and you need to stay away from sick people and out of the severe cold.

CHAPTER VII

RECIPES FOR LIFE

THE FIRST THING WE are going to talk about in this chapter is Nutrition.

Food Group	Daily Servings	Food and Serving size	other foods	Nutrients
Grains	7-8 daily

1 oz | ½ cup oatmeal

ready to eat cereal
1 slice whole wheat bread | whole wheat pita

Grain products | fiber

potassium |
| Vegetables | 4—5 daily | 6 oz Vegetable Juice

½ cup cooked
1 cup raw vegetables | Broccoli, carrots, collard greens potatoes, squash, tomatoes, sweet potatoes | fiber, magnesium,

potassium |

Fruits	4-5 daily	6 oz fruit juice	apricots, bananas	fiber,
		1 medium fruit	grapefruit, grapes, oranges,	magnesium,
		½ cups dried fruit	prunes, mangoes,	potassium
			peaches, pineapples,	
		½ cup fresh fruit	melons, strawberries	
Low fat Or fat free Dairy food		1 cup fat free milk	fat-free or low fat or reg frozen yogurt	iron, protein
		1 ½ oz low-fat or fat free cheese		
Meats,	No more than 2 per day	3 oz cooked meat	lean meat trimmed	magnesium, iron, protein
Poultry And Fish		poultry or fish baked not fried	fat trimmed skinless poultry	

Nuts, seeds or dried beans	4-5 a week	1/3 cup or 1 ½ oz nuts, or 2 Tbsp seeds	almonds, filberts, mixed nuts, peanuts sunflower seeds, kidney beans, lentils,	fiber, magnesium, potassium
Dry beans		1 cup cooked dry beans	peas	
Fat and Dash Diet Oils		1 Tbsp low fat soft margarine	Olive, corn, canola or sunflower oil	low in fat essential oils
		2 Tbsp low fat or fat free mayonnaise, or light or fat free salad dressing,		

There are listed twenty cuts of beef that meet the government labeling guidelines for lean, they are:

For 3 oz serving	grams saturated fat	grams of total fat
Eye or round steak	1.4	4.0
Sirloin tip side steak	1.6	4.1
Top round roast and steak	1.6	4.6
Bottom round roast and steak	1.7	4.9
Top sirloin steak	1.9	4.9
Brisket flat half	1.9	5.1
95% lean ground beef	2.4	5.1
Round tip roast	1.9	5.3
Round steak	1.9	5.3
Shank cross cuts	1.9	5.4
Chuck shoulder pot roast	1.8	5.7
Sirloin tip center roast and steak	2.1	5.8
Chuck shoulder steak	1.9	6.0
Bottom round steak (Western Griller)	2.2	6.0
Top loin (strip) steak	2.3	6.0
Shoulder petite tender and medallions	2.4	6.1
Flank steak	2.6	6.3
Shoulder cut (ranch) steak	2.4	6.5
Tri-tip roast and steak	2.6	7.1

Twenty cuts of beef meeting the government labeling guidelines for lean (continued)

Tenderloin roast and steak	2.7	7.1
T-bone steak	3.0	8.2
Compared to chicken:		
Skinless chicken breast	0.9	3.0
Skinless chicken thigh	2.6	9.2

Obviously the skinless chicken breast is the best of all of the cuts of meat listed above. For those of you who prefer dark meat the thigh even skinless is the worst of all of the above listed cuts of meat for you. But all do meet government guidelines for lean.

Lean: Less than 10gr of total fat and 4.5 or less of saturated fat and less than 95 mg of cholesterol per serving and per 100grams. Source: U.S. Department Agriculture, Agricultural Research Services, 2005. USDA Nutrient Database for Standard Research, Release18. Based on cooked servings, visible fat trimmed. See: **MyPyramid.gov**
Visit: "http://www.beefitsWhatsForDinner.com/" for more recipes and information about lean beef.
From 2005, Cattlemen's Beef Board and National Cattlemen's Association
USDA guidelines for a healthy diet state 60 grams of fat American Heart Association guidelines for cardiac diet is 30 grams of fat daily.

Eating out is a problem if you aren't careful, you should get a nutritional informational sheet from the restaurant that you intend to eat at they are required by federal law to provide that information for you. Don't be shy ask for it. Many restaurants will prepare foods to order so even if what you want isn't on the menu, you may still be able to get a healthy meal don't be afraid to ask. If your not sure about a particular restaurant, phone before you go. When you choose to go out for Mexican food or stop for a quick meal of Chinese food, you can find delicious, nutritious choices. To help find healthy foods when you eat out use the following tips. Cajun food is spicy. It originated in southern France but took hold in the predominantly French areas of southern Louisiana. Avoid fried seafood and hush puppies. Blackened entrees are usually saturated in butter or oil, covered with spices and pan fried; ask the cook to use only a small amount of oil. Ask for all gravies and sauces on the side. Try broiled crawfish or shrimp instead of fried, Creole and Jambalaya instead of gumbo, etouffe and sauces made with roux. Try broiled or grilled seafood instead of fried, white rice instead of dirty rice as it contains chicken gizzards, livers, butter etc.

Chinese foods choose entries with lost of vegetables, Chop suey with steamed rice is an example or substitute chicken for duck, when possible skip the crispy fried noodles. Try wonton or hot-and-sour soup instead of egg drop soup, steamed dumplings instead of egg rolls or fried wontons. Try broiled, boiled, steamed or lightly stir-fried entrees instead of deep fried entrees. Try dishes with lots of vegetables instead of dishes with fried meats, steamed rice instead of fried rice. Always ask if you can have your food prepared with out salt and bring with you a small shaker of sea salt mixed 50-50 with Morton salt substitute. Salt Substitute is potassium chloride, potassium being something that you are probably in need of.

Health foods avoid Granola made with oil substitute fat-free or low-fat granola, try salads with fat-free dressings instead of oil-based dressings, sandwiches with fat-free Miracle Whip or fat-free mayonnaise instead of regular mayonnaise or Miracle Whip, yogurt-based dishes made with fat-free yogurt instead of whole-egg dishes. Eat fat-free ice cream or low fat frozen yogurt like Brayers or Ben and Gerry's For these and other tips see the pamphlet from the AMA entitled Tips for Eating Out The best restaurant to eat at is Subway.

The following are the nutrition guidelines put out by the Subway restaurant and they fit very well into a 30 gram fat daily cardiac diet or 60 gram fat daily healthy diet.

6-inch Subs	Calories Fat	(grams)
Sweet Onion Chicken Teriyaki	370	5.0
Turkey Breast	280	4.5
Ham	290	5.0
Oven Roasted Chicken Breast	310	5.0
Club	320	6.0
Turkey Breast & Ham	290	5.0
Veggie Delight	230	3.0
Fit Mini Subs		
Ham	180	3.0
Roast Beef	190	3.5
Turkey breast	190	3.0
Salad Options (Dressing and croutons not included)		
Ham	120	3.0
Oven roasted chicken breast	140	2.5
Roast beef	120	3.0
Subway club	150	4.0
Sweet Onion Teriyaki	210	3.0
Turkey Breast	110	2.5

Turkey Breast and Ham	120	3.0
Veggie Delight	60	1.0

Toasted sandwiches and other favorites

Steak and cheese	400	12.0
Subway Melt	380	12.0

Double Stacked Sandwiches

Double Subway Club	420	8.0
Double		

Subway desserts That are under 10 grams of fat

Apple Slices (1 pkg.)	35	0.0
Oatmeal Raisin cookie	200	8.0
Raisins	130	0.0

Subways breeds

Italian (white) bread	200	2.0
Wheat bread	200	2.5
Italian Herb and Cheese	250	5.0
Honey Oat	250	3.5
Parmesan Oregano Bread	220	3.0
Hearty Italian Bread	220	2.0
Monterey Cheddar	240	5.0
Mini Italian (White) Bread	140	1.5
Mini Wheat Bread	140	2.0
Wrap	190	4.5

Subway Cheeses

American, Processed	40	3.5
Monterey Cheddar, Shredded	50	4.5

Subway Cheeses Continued

Natural Cheddar	60	5.0
Pepper jack	50	4.0

Provolone	50	4.0
Swiss	50	4.5

Subway Condiments, Sauces and Dressings

Bacon (2 Strips)	45	3.5
Banana Peppers (3 Slices)	0	0.0
Jalapeno Peppers (3 Slices)	0	0.0
Fat Free Honey Mustard Sauce	30	0.0
Fat Free Sweet Onion Sauce	40	0.0
Fat Free Red Wine Vinaigrette	30	0.0
Chipotle Southwest Sauce	100	10.0
Light Mayonnaise	50	5.0
Mayonnaise	110	12.0
Mustard-Yellow or Deli Brown	5	0.0
Olive Oil Blend	45	5.0
Ranch Dressing	120	13.0
Vinegar	0	0.0

Salad Dressings

Red Wine Vinaigrette	80	1.0
Fat Free Italian	35	0.0
Ranch	320	35.0
Subway has an excellent selection of chips		
Baked Lays	130	1.5
Baked Lays Cheddar and Sour Cream	140	3.5
Baked Lays Sour Cream and Onion	140	3.0
Baked Lays KC Masterpiece	140	3.0
Baked Lays NACHO CHEESIER	170	4.0
SUNCHIPS Harvest Cheddar	210	9.0
SUNCHIPS Original	210	9.0
Doritos Light NACHO CHEESIER	120	1.5

Lay's Light Original	75	0.0
Baked Ruffles Cheddar and Sour Cream	140	4.0

Keep in mind that when selecting your Subway lunch to select items that will allow you to remain under 60 grams of fat for the entire day or 30 grams of fat if you are on a cardiac diet.

Burger King has a few items that will keep you on your diet.

Whopper Jr. without Mayo	290	12
Fire Grilled Hamburger	290	12
Chicken Tenders 5 pc w/Sweet & Sour	255	12
Hamlette Breakfast sandwich	330	14
Tender Grilled Chicken Sandwich	450	10
Tender Grilled Chkn sandwich w/o Sauce	400	7
Side Salad w/Ken's Lite Italian Dressing	80	6

Burger King Desserts

Mott's Strawberry Flavored Applesauce	90	0.0

McDonalds Menu has improve and added some healthy Items

Original Hamburger	250	9
Original Cheeseburger	300	12
Premium Chicken Classic Grilled	420	10
Chicken nuggets 4 Pc	170	10
Ranch Snack wrap Grilled Chicken	270	10
Honey Mustard Snack Wrap Grld Chkn	260	9
Asian Salad with Grilled Chicken	300	10
Premium Bacon Ranch Salad w/Grld Chkn	260	9
Premium Caesar Salad w/Grld Chkn	220	6

Side Salad	20	0.0
Snack Size Fruit & Walnut Salad	210	8
Newman's own Balsamic Vinaigrette	40	3
Newman's own Low Fat Family Italian	60	2.5
Newman's own Low Fat Sesame Gngr	90	2.5
Breakfast at McDonald's		
Egg McMuffen	300	12
Hash Browns	140	8
McDonald's Desserts		
Apple Dippers	35	0.0
McDonald' Desserts Continued		
Low fat Caramel Dip	70	0.5
Fruit'n Yogurt Parfait without Granola	130	2
Fruit'n Yogurt Parfait	160	2
Vanilla Reduced Fat Ice Cream Cone	150	3.5
Strawberry Sundae	280	6
Caramel Sunday	340	8
Strawberry or Vanilla Shake	560	13
Baked Hot Apple Pie	270	12

Charley's Grilled Subs is one of my favorite places to eat,

Six Inch Subs		
Philly Steak Subs	300	14
Philly Chicken Sub	260	10
Grilled Chicken Subs	280	10
Grilled Deli Subs	410	9
Gourmet Fries	250	12
Grilled Salads	140	2.5

Charley's also has three of the best Natural Lemonades you'll ever taste Kiwi Lemonade, (My personal favorite) I would Drive 50 Miles one way for a cup. Raspberry Lemonade and Lemonade Ice Tea.

The first recipe for life
is for all of you guys and gals who love their
biscuits and gravy:

Ingredients:

Gravy;

1 two Quart sauce pan

2 Cups cold water

1 frozen turkey sausage patty or 1 Jimmie Dean reduced fat sausage patty (more flavor with Jimmie Dean)

1 Pkg McCormick's Sausage Gravy mix (taste as good as the best restaurant biscuits and gravy you ever ate)

Biscuits;

2 1/4 cups reduced fat bisquick

2/3 cup fat free milk

Preparation:

Gravy; Place sausage in saucepan and heat, chopping with spatula until fully cooked and in small pieces.

Place 2 cups cold water in saucepan with sausage and stir in sausage gravy mix with wire wisk until fully dissolved and smooth.

Turn heat on to medium and heat until thick almost to boil.

Biscuits and Gravy Continues

Biscuits:

Pour bisquick into large bowl

Mix until mixture turns loose from bowl. Roll dough out onto lightly floured surface and with floured hands need dough for 1 minute then start spreading dough out until it is even about a half inch thick. Next with biscuit cutter or a small glass that is about the size around that you want your biscuits cut the biscuits and place on cookie sheet or pizza pan. Cook biscuits at 425 until brown on outside.

Now you are ready to enjoy a beautiful and delicious biscuit and gravy break fast and if you limit yourself to one biscuit with gravy you are only eating about 7 grams of fat 6 if you use the straight turkey sausage.

Peanut Butter Sandwiches

If you are like me you grew up eating a peanut butter sandwich for lunch most of the time. I missed my peanut butter sandwich and glass of cold milk. Good news, you don't have to give it up just change to reduced fat JIF and eat 1 tablespoon of peanut butter on a slice of Roman Meal bread and you will be getting about 12 grams of fat. But remember only one per day. Drink a glass of cold fat free milk with your sandwich and it will taste like heaven after eating the hospital cardiac diet for a week or so. After surgery and that week of cardiac diet you will never miss the old peanut butter or the old milk. If you haven't been on the cardiac diet yet because you haven't had a heart attack or open heart surgery or a heart catheterization. Now is the time that you need to start this diet. Get use to the taste of the lower fat items unless you just like people opening you up like a can of sardines and playing with your heart and other organs. If you will eat these fat free items that I am outlining after a month you won't know the difference between them and the stuff loaded with fat.

Bacon and Eggs:

What about bacon and eggs. Well get yourself a microwave bacon tray and no more than once a month microwave your bacon crisp and dump out the bacon grease because you'll never be able to use it again. Spray a skillet with PAM cooking spray and fry your Eggland's Best eggs the way you like them. Serve them with Roman Meal Bread toast with your favorite jelly or jam. Hear we have a breakfast of less than 12 grams of fat, but its all the bad kind of fat, so don't do this more than about once a month.

Now what about if you want something beside cereal for breakfast and you had your bacon and eggs last week. Well have yourself a scrambled egg or vegetarian omelet.

Ingredients:

> 1 carton of Eggbeaters which are 99% real egg
> with no cholesterol and fat = 2 eggs
> Or you can use Egglands Best

Chopped garlic and chopped onions

½ tsp Morton salt substitute (potassium chloride)

Or ½ tsp sea salt or a mixture of the two

Green peppers chopped

Fat free shredded cheddar cheese made by Kraft. The Kraft fat free cheese taste great it just isn't a sharp cheddar. Kraft also makes fat free cheddar slices and fat free Pepper Jack slices that are not to bad.

Salsa or other topping if desired

Preparation:

Spray hot skillet with PAM cooking spray

Pour Egg Beaters into skillet

Add onions and small amount of garlic

Add green peppers

Last add shredded cheese

Fold omelet together

Place on plate and add salsa if desired

(you can add cooked chopped turkey or vegetable sausage)

Scrambled Eggs or Vegetarian Omelet:

Ingredients:

1 carton of Eggbeaters which are 99% real eggs without cholesterol and fat = 2 eggs

Chopped garlic and chopped onions

½ tsp Morton Salt Substitute (potassium Chloride)

Or Sea salt or a 50-50 mixture of the two

Green peppers chopped

Fat free shredded cheddar cheese made by Kraft

The Kraft fat free cheeses taste great it just isn't an extra sharp cheese Kraft also makes fat free cheddar and Pepper Jack slices that are very good.

Salsa or other topping if desired.

Preparation:

Spray hot skillet with PAM cooking spray

Pour Egg Beaters into skillet

Add onions and small amount of garlic

Add green peppers

Last add shredded cheese

Fold omelet together

Place on plate and add salsa if desired

(you can add cooked chopped turkey, vegetable or deer sausage).

Salmon Patties;
are always great and a vital part of a good cardiac diet:

Ingredients:

1 large can of Salmon (your choice of brands and type)

1 carton of Eggbeaters = 2 eggs about 12 fat free soda crackers crumbed seasoning such as garlic powder and onion powder chopped garlic and chopped onions can also be used ½ tsp Morton salt

½ tsp black pepper

1 large skillet or griddle

1 Can PAM cooking spray

Preparation:

In large bowl mix all ingredients, knead until Thoroughly mixed into good consistency for Making patties. Make into patties.

Spray griddle or skillet with PAM

Fry patties until golden brown

Serving suggestions:

Serving size 1 salmon patty.

Start with a salad with fat free ranch dressing (receipt to follow) or other fat free dressings that you prefer. Serve with green beans cooked with a generous helping of imitation bacon bits and seasoned to taste with above seasoning or substitute spinach and add 1 tablespoon of vinegar. A helping of garlic mash potatoes made with fat free milk. Substitution of cheesy mash potatoes make with fat free cheddar cheese is also good. For desert a nice bowl of mixed fruit or a fruit salad.

Fat Free Ranch Dressing:

Ingredients:

One packed of Hidden Valley Ranch Dip Mix

I cup of Fat Free Miracle Whip Salad Dressing

I cup of cold Fat Free Skim Milk

Preparation:

In a bowl or large measuring cup mix all ingredients

Together with a blender until smooth and creamy looking.

Your taste buds will love it and your heart will thank you.

Tuna Salad:

2 Can (6oz each) Tuna, Water Pack

1/3 green onions chopped

6 ½ Tbsp Fat Free Mirical Whip Salad Dressing

4 Medium Sweat Pickles Chopped

I. Drain Tuna for 5 minutes. Break apart with fork.

2. Add Onions and Mirical Whip and Sweat Pickles, Mix Well

3. Serve on Multigrain Bread such as Roman Meal Bread

Makes: 5 Servings

Serving Size: ½ Cups

Each serving Provides:

Calories: 146

Total Fat: 7 g

Saturated Fat: I g

Cholesterol:	25 mg
Sodium:	158 mg
Total Fiber:	1 g
Protein:	16 g
Carbohydrates:	4g
Potassium:	201 mg

Shrimp Scampi:

Ingredients:

Raw shrimp, pealed tail on

Olive oil

Oregano

Italian Seasoning

Garlic (Powdered, Chopped or grated)

Onion (Powered or chopped)

1 Tablespoon Mustard

Preparation:

Amount of shrimp depends on number to be served 1 Bag medium shrimp serves about 4.

Heat Olive Oil (Amount depends on amount of shrimp to be cooked, must be enough to cover shrimp.

Add seasoning about 1 tablespoon each

Add onion about ¼ cup

Add garlic about 1 Tablespoon

Add mustard

Add Shrimp cook on medium heat until Shrimp are pink.

Serve in small bowl with some of the olive oil in the bowl.

Serving suggestions: Serve with salad and fat free ranch dressing and garlic toast use Promise Heart Healthy Margarine.

Spaghetti:

Ingredients:

Good quality spaghetti such as American Beauty or Barilla (try the whole grain spaghetti)

½ Lb 96% ground beef or ground deer meat.

1 teaspoon of onion powder

1 Tablespoon oregano

1 Tablespoon Italian seasoning

1-3 drops peppermint extract (flavor enhancer does not make taste pepperminty).

Homemade Turkey Sausage:

For 16	For 48	Cut 16 or 48 10" squares of freezer wrap or wax paper
2lbs	6lbs	extra lean ground turkey breast*
1 tsp	1 Tbls	black pepper
1 ½ tsp	1 ½ Tbls	dried sage
1 ½ tsp	1 ½ Tbls	dried thyme

1 ½ tsp	1 ½ Tbls	dried rosemary
¼ tsp	1 tsp	red pepper flakes
¼ tsp	1 tsp	cayenne pepper
10 grinds	30 grinds	fresh ground black pepper
¾ tsp	2 tsp	sea salt or McCormick's salt substitute
1 Tbls	3 Tbls	oil (canola or Olive)
¾ cup	2 ¼ cups	applesauce, unsweetened

Preparation:

Mix ingredients together very thoroughly using your hands if necessary. (wash them thoroughly first)

Divide the sausage mixture into 4 equal portions in the bowl.

From each portion, make 4 (small batch) or 12 (large batch) 2" balls. Place each ball on the center of a wax paper square.

Fold the square up from the bottom, the sides and then the top.

This will flatten the ball into a patty.

Place 4 or 8 patties each in a freezer bag an freeze.

To Cook:

Coat a large nonstick skillet with cooking spray. Place on medium-high heat.

Unwrap frozen patties (no need to thaw) and place in skillet.

Cook patties **6** minutes on each side (less if not frozen) until no longer pink inside (do not overcook or they will be dry).

Serve with scrambled Egg Beaters or fried Eggland's best eggs fried with PAM and serve with toast.

*Deer meat can be substituted and if grinding turkey yourself, use either a cutter for fine or course sausage, depending on your preference.

Rainbow Fruit Salad:

I Large Mango, Peeled, diced

2c Fresh Blueberries

2 bananas, sliced

2c Fresh Strawberries, halved

2 Nectarines, unpeeled, sliced

I Kiwi fruit, peeled, sliced

Honey-orange sauce:

1/3 c Unsweetened orange juice

2 Tsp Lemon juice

I ½ Honey

¼ tsp Ground Ginger

Dash Nutmeg

1. Prepare the fruit

2. Combine all ingredients for sauce and mix

3. Just before serving, pour

   Honey-Orange Sauce on fruit

Yeild: 12 servings

Serving size:4-oz cup

Each Serving Provides

Calories: 96

Total Fat: I g

Saturated Fat: >I g

Cholesterol: 0 mg

Sodium: 4 mg

Total fiber: 3 g

Protein: I g

Carbohydrates: 24 g

Potassium: 302 mg

BAY SCALLOP KABOBS

3	Medium green peppers, cut into 1 ½ in squares
1 ½ lb	Fresh bay Scallops
1 pt	Cherry tomatoes
¼ C	Dry white wine
¼ C	Vegetable oil or olive oil
3 Tbsp	Lemon juice
Dash	Garlic powder
To taste	Black pepper
4	Skewers

1. Parboil green peppers for 2 minutes
2. Alternately thread first three
   ingredients on skewers.
3. Combine next 5 ingredients.
4. Brush kabobs with wine/oil/lemon
Mixture, then place on grill (or under
5. Grill for 15 minutes,
Broiler).
Turning and basting
Frequently.

Yield : 4 Servings
Serving Size:1 Kabob

(6 oz)
Each serving provides
Calories: 224
Total fat: 6 g
Saturated fat: 1
Cholesterol: 43 mg
Sodium: 335 mg
Total fiber: 3 g
Protein: 30 g
Carbohydrates: 13 g
Potassium: 993 mg

Banana Mousse

2 Tbsp	fat free milk
4 tsp	sugar
1 tsp	vanilla

1	medium banana, cut in quarters
1 C	plain low fat yogurt
8 slices	(¼ inch each) banana

1. Place milk, sugar, vanilla and banana in blender
Process for 15 seconds at high speed until smooth.

2. Pour mixture into small bowl and
   fold in yogurt. Chill.

3. Spoon into four dessert dishes and
   garnish each with two
Banana slices just before serving.

Yield: 4 servings

Serving size: ½ cup

Each serving provides

Calories: 94

Total fat: 1 g

Saturated fat: 1 g

Cholesterol: 4 mg

Sodium: 47 mg

Total fiber: 1 g

Protein: 1 g

Carbohydrates: 18 g

Potassium: 297 mg

Chocolate Angel Food Cake with Cherries:

16 oz package angel food cake mix

1/3 cup unsweetened cocoa powder

½ teaspoon ground cinnamon

1 cup frozen fat-free whipped topping, thawed

4 cups fresh pitted bing cherries

1. In large mixing bowl, stir together the cake mix,

Cocoa powder and cinnamon. Prepare the cake

Package direction.

2. To serve, top each slice of cake with a dollop of

Whipped topping and cherries

Each serving provides	
Calories:	130
Protein:	0.5 grams
Carbohydrates	29 grams
Total fat:	0.5 grams
Sat. fat	0 grams
Cholesterol:	0 grams
Fiber:	3 grams
Sodium	171 mg

Hot and smokey Chipotle-Garlic Dip:

Serves	8; 2 Tablespoons per serving
2/3	fat-free or light sour cream
3	Tablespoons fat-free or light Mayonnaise or Miracle Whip
2-3	Tablespoons fat-free milk
2	Tablespoons fresh lemon juice
1	Chipotle pepper, canned in adobo sauce
1	medium garlic clove, minced
1/8	teaspoon sea salt fresh cilantro sprigs

In a food processor or blender, process all the ingredients except the cilantro until smooth. To serve, transfer the dip to a serving bowl. Garnish with the cilantro.

Calories	44	Carbohydrates	6 g
Total Fat	1.0 g	Fiber	0 g
Saturated	0.0 g	Sugars	2 g
polyunsaturated	0.0 g	roteins	2 g
Monounsaturated	0.0 g	Calcium	33 g
Cholesterol	5.0 g	Potassium	54 g
Sodium	152 mg		

Creamy Cole Slaw

Serves 7; ½ cup per serving

Slaw

1	10-ounce package shredded cabbage (8-9 cups)
½	cup chopped onion
½	large green bell pepper, sliced into thin strips
1	medium carrot, shredded

Dressing

3-4	Tablespoons sugar
3	Tablespoons white vinegar
3 ½	Tablespoons water
2 ½	Tablespoons Fat-Free Miracle Whip
	Pepper to taste

In a large bowl, stir together the slaw ingredients. In a small bowl, whisk together the dressing ingredients. Pour over the slaw. Toss thoroughly. Cover and refrigerate for at least 1 hour before serving, in possible, to let the flavor blend.

Calories	73	Carbohydrates	12 g
Total Fat	0.0 g	Fiber	1 g
Saturated	0.0 g	Sugars	10 g
Polyunsaturated	1.0 g	Protein	1 g
Monounsaturated	2.0 g	Calcium	26 mg
Cholesterol	0 mg	Potassium	164 mg
Sodium	14 mg		

Other recipes and helps can be found in pamphlets published by the American Heart Association.

"Nutritious Nibbles"

"Shake Your Salt Habit"

"Tips For Eating Out"

"Just Move"

"About Your Bypass Surgery"